T0259599

# Clinical Issues and Affirmative Treatment with Transgender Clients

*Editors*

LYNNE CARROLL
LAUREN MIZOCK

# PSYCHIATRIC CLINICS OF NORTH AMERICA

www.psych.theclinics.com

March 2017 • Volume 40 • Number 1

ELSEVIER

1600 John F. Kennedy Boulevard • Suite 1800 • Philadelphia, Pennsylvania, 19103-2899

http://www.theclinics.com

PSYCHIATRIC CLINICS OF NORTH AMERICA Volume 40, Number 1
March 2017 ISSN 0193-953X, ISBN-13: 978-0-323-50985-5

Editor: Lauren Boyle
Developmental Editor: Kristen Helm

*Psychiatric Clinics of North America* (ISSN 0193-953X) is published quarterly by Elsevier Inc., 360 Park Avenue South, New York, NY 10010-1710. Months of issue are March, June, September, and December. Business and Editorial Offices: 1600 John F. Kennedy Blvd., Suite 1800, Philadelphia, PA 19103-2899. Periodicals postage paid at New York, NY and additional mailing offices. Subscription prices are $303.00 per year (US individuals), $628.00 per year (US institutions), $100.00 per year (US students/residents), $369.00 per year (Canadian individuals), $460.00 per year (international individuals), $791.00 per year (Canadian & international institutions), and $220.00 per year (Canadian & international students/residents). Foreign air speed delivery is included in all *Clinics'* subscription prices. All prices are subject to change without notice. **POSTMASTER:** Send address changes to *Psychiatric Clinics of North America*, Elsevier Health Sciences Division, Subscription Customer Service, 3251 Riverport Lane, Maryland Heights, MO 63043. **Customer Service: 1-800-654-2452 (US). From outside the United States, call 1-314-447-8871. Fax: 1-314-447-8029. E-mail: journalscustomerservice-usa@elsevier.com (for print support) and journalsonline support-usa@elsevier.com (for online support)**.

*Reprints.* For copies of 100 or more, of articles in this publication, please contact the Commercial Reprints Department, Elsevier Inc., 360 Park Avenue South, New York, New York 10010-1710. Tel.: 212-633-3874, Fax: 212-633-3820, E-mail: reprints@elsevier.com.

*Psychiatric Clinics of North America* is covered in *MEDLINE/PubMed (Index Medicus), Current Contents/Social and Behavioral Sciences, Social Science Citation Index, Embase/Excerpta Medica,* and PsycINFO.

# Contributors

## EDITORS

**LYNNE CARROLL, PhD, ABPP**
Professor of Psychology (Retired), Department of Psychology, University of North Florida; Psychologist, Independent Practice, Jacksonville, Florida

**LAUREN MIZOCK, PhD**
Doctoral Faculty, Fielding Graduate University, Clinical Psychology PhD Program; Psychologist, Private Practice, San Francisco, California

## AUTHORS

**EDWARD J. ALESSI, PhD, LCSW**
Assistant Professor, School of Social Work, Rutgers, The State University of New Jersey, Newark, New Jersey

**ASHLEY AUSTIN, PhD, LCSW**
Associate Professor, Director of the Center for Human Rights and Social Justice, School of Social Work, Barry University, Miami Shores, Florida

**STEPHANIE L. BUDGE, PhD**
Assistant Professor, University of Wisconsin-Madison, Madison, Wisconsin

**LYNNE CARROLL, PhD, ABPP**
Professor of Psychology (Retired), Department of Psychology, University of North Florida; Psychologist, Independent Practice, Jacksonville, Florida

**DEBORAH COOLHART, PhD, LMFT**
Assistant Professor, Department of Marriage and Family Therapy, Syracuse University, Syracuse, New York

**SHELLEY L. CRAIG, PhD, LCSW**
Associate Professor, Factor Inwentash Faculty of Social Work, University of Toronto, Toronto, Ontario, Canada

**MADELINE B. DEUTSCH, MD, MPH**
Associate Professor of Clinical and Family Community Medicine, Department of Family & Community Medicine, Center of Excellence for Transgender Health, University of California - San Francisco, San Francisco, California

**LORE M. DICKEY, PhD**
Assistant Professor, Department of Educational Psychology, Northern Arizona University, Flagstaff, Arizona

**LAURA ERICKSON-SCHROTH, MD, MA**
Assistant Professor, Comprehensive Psychiatric Emergency Program, Mount Sinai Beth Israel; Psychiatrist, Hetrick-Martin Institute, New York, New York

**KARA M. FITZGERALD, PhD**
Neuropsychologist, Department of Psychology, Lemuel Shattuck Hospital, Jamaica Plain, Massachusetts

**LIN FRASER, EdD, MFT, LPCC**
WPATH Past President; Private Practice, San Francisco, California

**RYAN NICHOLAS GORTON, MD**
Lyon-Martin Health Services, San Francisco, California; Adjunct Assistant Professor, Touro University of California, College of Osteopathic Medicine, Vallejo, California

**NICHOLAS C. HECK, PhD**
Department of Psychology, Marquette University, Milwaukee, Wisconsin

**COLTON L. KEO-MEIER, PhD**
Clinical Psychologist, Department of Psychology, University of Houston, Lee and Joe Jamail Specialty Care Center, Houston, Texas; Menninger Department of Psychiatry and Behavioral Sciences, Baylor College of Medicine, Houston, Texas; School of Medicine, University of Texas Medical Branch, Galveston, Texas

**GAIL KNUDSON, MD, MEd, FRCPC**
WPATH President; Clinical Associate Professor, Faculty of Medicine, University of British Columbia, Victoria, British Columbia, Canada

**LAUREN MIZOCK, PhD**
Doctoral Faculty, Fielding Graduate University, Clinical Psychology PhD Program; Psychologist, Private Practice, San Francisco, California

**DARAN L. SHIPMAN, MA, LMFT**
Adjunct Faculty, Department of Marriage and Family Therapy, Syracuse University, Syracuse, New York

**ANNELIESE A. SINGH, PhD**
Department of Counseling & Human Development Services, The University of Georgia, Athens, Georgia

**DANIEL WALINSKY, PhD**
Psychology Department, Salem State University, Salem, Massachusetts

**LINDA M. WESP, MSN, FNP-C**
Jonas Nurse Leaders Scholar, College of Nursing, University of Wisconsin-Milwaukee, Milwaukee, Wisconsin

# Contents

and mental health with minimal adverse effects. Ongoing research is needed to improve understanding about specific risks of hormone therapy and surgical outcomes.

Families of transgender and gender-nonconforming youth often seek therapy for assistance in understanding, accepting, and supporting their child. This article describes a gender-affirmative approach to family therapy and outlines strategies for addressing common challenges faced by the families of transgender and gender-nonconforming youth. Therapy begins by assessing family attunement and working with parents, siblings, and other family members to better support the youth. Once family attunement is achieved, therapy can begin to explore options for gender expression and/or transition. The therapeutic model is illustrated by applying it to case examples.

Research demonstrates that transgender and nonconforming (TGNC) elders face social isolation and discrimination in policies and practices in mental and health care settings. The purpose of this article is to provide clinicians with practical input about therapeutic issues and interventions for use with TGNC elders. A case vignette describes the challenges and rewards of therapy with an elder trans woman. Her story illustrates the complex interplay between age, life phase, and sociocultural and historical contexts. Recommendations regarding research, practice, and advocacy are offered.

Although there is growing awareness in contemporary society regarding transgender and gender nonconforming (TGNC) identities, transgender people continue to be highly marginalized and subject to transphobic discrimination and victimization. As a result, authentically expressing and navigating a TGNC identity can be difficult. Psychiatrists and other mental health professionals can play a key role in supporting TGNC client health and well-being through the use of trans-affirmative approaches. Trans-affirmative practice recognizes all experiences of gender as equally healthy and valuable. This article focuses on transgender affirmative cognitive behavior therapy.

Although there are descriptions of transgender-affirmative group psychotherapy services in the literature, there is limited research on the topic.

Mental health professionals who plan to offer such services should draw on evidence-based treatments, where appropriate, and have a working knowledge of current standards of care, practice guidelines, and counseling competencies. This article reviews and synthesizes the existing research and scholarship on this topic, placing an emphasis on group-specific competencies and intervention components that can be integrated into psychotherapy groups for transgender and gender nonconforming clients.

# PSYCHIATRIC CLINICS OF NORTH AMERICA

---

**RELATED INTEREST**

*Pediatric Clinics of North America*, December 2016 (Vol. 63, No. 6)
**Lesbian, Gay, Bisexual, and Transgender Youth**
Stewart L. Adelson, Nadia L. Dowshen, Harvey J. Makadon, and Robert Garofalo, *Editors*
Available at: http://www.pediatric.theclinics.com/

---

**THE CLINICS ARE AVAILABLE ONLINE!**
Access your subscription at:
www.theclinics.com

# Preface

# Trans-affirmative Care: Moving from Trans Allies To Trans Activists

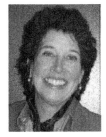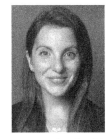

Lynne Carroll, PhD, ABPP    Lauren Mizock, PhD
*Editors*

"Clinical Issues and Affirmative Treatment with Transgender Clients" offers an up-to-date toolkit for clinical use with transgender and gender-diverse clients (TGD). The contributing authors represent diverse gender identities and sexual orientations. We also include a broad range of professional identities and affiliations—social workers, mental health counselors, psychologists, and physicians. Collectively, we embrace a trans-affirmative treatment paradigm that celebrates the broad spectrum of gender identities and the range of treatment options and outcomes.

We, the editors of this special issue, are cisgender. Our gender privilege and unearned advantages impact the research and clinical work that we do, and we must stay vigilant to our blindspots and biases. Our TGD colleagues have trained us and many other cisgender people in trans-affirmative care and research so that we do not rely on the trans community to conduct this work alone. Mental health providers must become trans-affirmative in their practice in order to better serve the trans community instead of expecting them to instruct us in their care. As cisgender people, we can move beyond the position of "trans ally" to "trans activist" in the mission to challenge transphobia[1] and recognize that we have gendered identities implicated in and affected by gender-based oppression.

While our collective consciousness about gender diversity shifts, and professional clinical guidelines and practices are revised, much work remains. Many clinicians report a lack of confidence, knowledge, and competence in trans-affirmative practice. Empirically supported treatments, longitudinal research, appropriate assessments, and models of clinical decision-making are needed.

The U.S. elected administration of 2017 threatens the rights of transgender people, including the support of conversion therapy, limitations to bathroom use, and allowing

Psychiatr Clin N Am 40 (2017) xi–xiii
http://dx.doi.org/10.1016/j.psc.2016.12.001
0193-953X/17/© 2016 Published by Elsevier Inc.

businesses to refuse service to trans people.² Consequently, we lead this special issue with dickey and Singh's article on social justice and advocacy. A political history of the relationship between TGD and the mental health communities is provided, and they outline the role of helping professionals in advocating for the rights of TGD people.

Fraser and Knudson provide insights as past and current presidents, respectively, of the World Professional Association for Transgender Health and explore challenges in the development of the Standards of Care for the Health of Transsexual, Transgender, and Gender Nonconforming People, Version 7 (SOC 7).

Mizock demonstrates how the increased prevalence of mental disorders among transgender individuals is largely impacted by transphobia, including suicidality, anxiety, depression, and other disorders.

dickey, Singh, and Walinsky focus on the treatment of trauma and nonsuicidal self-injury in transgender adults, with an emphasis on understanding the impact of gender minority stress on these problems.

Keo-Meier and Fitzgerald provide a much-needed overview of psychological testing and neurocognitive assessment with transgender adults, including the cognitive effects of hormone therapy on mood and cognition as well as personality and psychopathology assessments.

Budge and dickey address common but challenging clinical representations to help readers understand the nuances associated with writing letters and engaging in consultation with interdisciplinary health care providers.

Gorton and Erickson-Schroth as well as Wesp and Deutsch adopt an individualized approach to gender-affirming hormonal and surgical treatment of TGD persons based upon current professional guidelines and research regarding the use of hormones and gender-affirming surgical options.

Coolhart and Shipman provide an in-depth description of their gender-affirmative family therapy model, which attends to ways that clinicians can increase family's understanding and support of their child's gender expression and transition options.

Carroll discusses therapeutic issues and interventions for use with TGD elders. A case vignette is offered to illustrate the complex interplay between age, life phase, and sociocultural and historical contexts.

Austin, Craig, and Alessi present their model, Transgender Affirmative-Cognitive Behavior Therapy, to help TGD clients identify and challenge transphobic attitudes and behaviors and internalized stigma in a safe and supportive environment.

Heck provides a compelling rationale for the use of group counseling as a treatment modality and identifies specific professional guidelines and competencies necessary to provide trans-affirmative group psychotherapy.

In closing, we extend our gratitude to lore dickey, PhD for helping to develop this special issue in the initial stages. We should also note that language and word choice when working with the trans community is constantly evolving, and you may find differences in the use of terms such as gender nonconforming or gender diverse depending on the author. We hope you find the contents of this special issue helpful in filling the gaps in research, assessment, and psychotherapy with TGD individuals and families.

Lynne Carroll, PhD, ABPP
1810 Sevilla Boulevard #308
Atlantic Beach, FL 32233, USA

Lauren Mizock, PhD
3610 Sacramento Street
San Francisco, CA 94118, USA

E-mail addresses:
lcarroll1258@gmail.com (L. Carroll)
Lauren.mizock@gmail.com (L. Mizock)

**REFERENCES**

1. Mizock L, Page K. Evaluating the ally role: social justice and collective action in counseling and psychology. J Soc Action Couns Psychol 2016;8(1):17–33.
2. Stack L. Trump victory alarms gay and lesbian groups. New York Times 2016. Available at: http://www.nytimes.com/2016/11/11/us/politics/trump-victory-alarms-gay-and-transgender-groups.html?_r=0.

# Social Justice and Advocacy for Transgender and Gender-Diverse Clients

 CrossMark

lore m. dickey, PhD[a],*, Anneliese A. Singh, PhD[b]

## KEYWORDS

- Transgender • Gender diverse • Advocacy • Social justice

## KEY POINTS

- Mental health providers are well-positioned to serve as advocates for transgender and gender-diverse people.
- Mental health providers must have a good working knowledge of the history of their relationship to the transgender and gender-diverse (TGD) community.
- Professional organizations have developed policy statements that support the role of the provider as advocate.

Many scholars have called on counseling and psychological services for increased attention to social justice and advocacy when working with transgender and gender-diverse (TGD) clients.[1,2] These calls for attention to social justice and advocacy are supported by research documenting extensive health disparities and discrimination among TGD people in society.[3–6] TGD people experience high rates of not only vulnerability to societal discrimination and violence, but also high rates of negative health outcomes related to these experiences, such as suicide,[7] depression, anxiety,[8] and substance abuse.[9]

In addition, counseling and psychological professional associations have joined these calls for mental health practitioners to engage in social justice change within the helping professions. The American Counseling Association (ACA) adopted counseling competencies with transgender clients in 2010.[10] These competencies

Disclosure Statement: Neither of the authors have a conflict of interest nor are we receiving any funding for this work.

[a] Department of Educational Psychology, Northern Arizona University, 801 South Knoles Drive, Building 27A, Room 110, PO Box 5774, Flagstaff, AZ 86011-5774, USA; [b] Department of Counseling & Human Development Services, The University of Georgia, 402 Aderhold Hall, Athens, GA 30602-7142, USA
* Corresponding author.
E-mail address: lore.dickey@nau.edu

Psychiatr Clin N Am 40 (2017) 1–13
http://dx.doi.org/10.1016/j.psc.2016.10.009
0193-953X/17/© 2016 Elsevier Inc. All rights reserved.

described eight areas of training where counselors could engage in social justice change when working with transgender clients:

1. Human growth and development
2. Social and cultural foundations
3. Helping relationships
4. Group work
5. Professional orientation
6. Career and lifestyle development
7. Assessment
8. Research and program evaluation

The American Psychological Association also developed guidelines for psychological practice with transgender and gender nonconforming clients,[11] where attention to issues of societal equity with transgender clients was detailed with 16 guidelines within five domains: (1) foundational knowledge and awareness; (2) stigma, discrimination, and barriers to care; (3) lifespan development; (4) assessment, therapy, and intervention; and (5) research, education, and training.

The World Professional Association of Transgender Health (WPATH)[12] also has begun to more explicitly examine the importance of social change efforts that increase awareness, respect, and dignity of TGD people.

One of the major challenges to engaging in social justice and advocacy is that mental health professionals may not always be aware of the history of counseling and psychology that TGD people have with health care. In this article, the sociopolitical and historical context of mental health care is discussed. In addition, the professional role of advocacy is also discussed in relation to the major professional documents described previously when engaging in social change. Finally, specific recommendations for social justice and advocacy strategies are provided.

Advocacy and social justice are related but distinct terms. Advocacy is related to the ways in which providers take action in support of their client's needs.[2] This might include working with school administrators, employers, or providers to ensure that the individual has access to the necessary resources and services to support their affirmed gender. Social justice is similar in that it also targets the needs of marginalized people. However, it is more of a theoretic approach to clinical work.[13] Social justice approaches recognize the systemic barriers that client's face and work to dismantle oppression.

## HISTORY OF THE ADVOCACY MOVEMENT FOR GENDER-DIVERSE PEOPLE

Recent advocacy for transgender people began in the 1990s around two different issues. The first issue was related to trans people's identities. No longer were TGD[a] people hiding in closets and blending in with the woodwork. Instead, we were holding our heads high and celebrating our gender in all of the ways and varieties that we were able to display. The second issue of advocacy, which remains a deep concern for TGD people, was the ways in which our stories were erased in the "war against AIDS." TGD people are adversely affected by human immunodeficiency virus (HIV)/AIDS and often erased when it comes time for care. Trans women who were affected

---

[a] In this article the authors use transgender and gender diverse (TGD) as a broadly inclusive manner of identifying transgender people. Recently, the term transgender and gender nonconforming has been used; however, the authors believe this term can have the effect of pathologizing one's gender identity and expression because gender is on a spectrum and has existed throughout history.

by HIV were lumped into public health statistics listing them as men who have sex with men. Although there were some similarities in the ways in which they engaged with each other in the community, the similarities disappeared fairly quickly after that.

In recent years, some have said that transgender rights represent unmet civil rights. We will not argue the veracity of that statement, but certainly agree with the sentiment that there is much work to do to provide TGD people with safe places live, access to medical care, and other basic human rights. Before we move forward to address these pressing needs, we must look back to explore the history that brought us to this place.

The lives of TGD people have been visible across history and on all continents around the world. Similar to the erasure of TGD lives during the HIV crisis, indigenous peoples with gender diverse identities have been erased from the cultural history as the result of colonization. This erasure has led to the reinforcement of the gender binary. Any persons who live outside the gender binary are considered to be invisible. Their gender does not fit with the boxes that society has fixed and therefore they are not, and likely cannot, be safe in expressing their true identity. As a result, TGD people have been relegated to positions of poverty and some have been, and continue to be, criminalized. Any person who is forced to live on the streets, wrongly fired from their jobs, or evicted by their landlord is likely to struggle to ensure their most basic needs are met (eg, food, clothing, and shelter). Images of these people are not what make the morning news; rather, images or reports of people being incarcerated for supposed sex or drug crimes make the news. That TGD people are portrayed in this negative light leads to more erasure of TGD people's lives.

For TGD people to be safe, many changes must be made with regard to basic civil and human rights. As of the writing of this article, there has been a tidal wave of change. It is unclear whether those changes will persist over time. The Obama administration has implemented several regulations and executive orders that effectively protect TGD people (eg, nondiscrimination protection for federal employees and contractors, protection for TGD students in the education setting). In addition to these executive orders, TGD people in some US states are protected from discrimination in housing, employment, and public accommodation. These rights are far from universal. Additionally, it seems that each time some progress is made to protect the lives of TGD people, legislation is proposed that not only strips away those rights but also pathologizes and criminalizes TGD people. A recent example of this is the so-called "bathroom bill." These bills require a person to use a bathroom based on the sex they were assigned at birth or the sex that is listed on their birth certificate. Proponents of these measures claim that women and children are at risk of sexual predators in public restrooms if TGD people are allowed to use a restroom that is consistent with their affirmed gender identity. What these proponents fail to also mention is the numbers of times that TGD people are assaulted or harassed in public places. More often, TGD people's lives are in jeopardy because TGD people often face acts of violence in public restrooms.

Changes have also occurred in other realms. There is beginning to be greater access to research funding and large data sets that are inclusive of TGD people. Although federal surveillance data are not yet inclusive of demographic questions that allow TGD people to be "counted," such organizations as the National Center for Transgender Equality have conducted two large-scale studies exploring discrimination. With regard to research funding, the federal government continues to fund research into HIV, which is often inclusive of TGD women. Additionally, there are some national research projects underway that will take a broad, affirming approach to understanding the lived experiences of TGD people. It is possible that an important tipping point has been reached with regard to this work and that large government research projects will be required to collect demographic data about TGD people so that policy decisions can accurately reflect the challenges faced by TGD people.

Another recent change was the lifting of the ban that prohibited TGD people from openly serving in the US military. Lesbian, gay, and bisexual people were allowed to openly serve when Don't Ask, Don't Tell[b] was overturned, but this regulation change was not inclusive of TGD people.[14] In July of 2016, the US military lifted the ban against TGD people.[15] As a result, TGD people are allowed to openly serve in the military, similar to their lesbian, gay, and bisexual counterparts. Like other such changes, it may be some time before the day-to-day workings of the military catch up with the regulations.

Mental health providers have their own history of negatively impacting the lives of TGD people. Historically, mental health providers have taken a role that was seen by TGD people as being a gatekeeper.[16] In some cases, TGD people were not provided access to necessary transition-related care. As a result, TGD people learned to tell their providers the "right" story to ensure that they would be provided access to care.[11] Fortunately, the need for these similar stories has mostly fallen away and there is greater recognition and celebration of the variation in TGD people's identity trajectories.[11,12] Like mental health providers, medical providers also have a complicated history with TGD patients. This is in part because medical providers are the ones who require letters for the commencement of a medical transition. In addition to this requirement, TGD people's lives have been unnecessarily medicalized. Social justice, as a theoretic approach, and advocacy, as an active intervention, can serve to enhance the lives of TGD people. The next section addresses the role of helping professionals in the areas of social justice and advocacy.

## ROLE OF HELPING PROFESSIONALS

Helping professionals play a key role in advancing the rights of TGD people. This section explores the roles of various professional organizations including the WPATH, the American Psychological Association, the ACA, and the American Psychiatric Association. Each organization has several ways in which they may engage in advocacy and social justice. They have all been involved in advancing affirmative care for TGD people through policy statements, amicus briefs, and legislative advocacy to name a few.

### *World Professional Association for Transgender Health*

The WPATH has a mission that includes the need to advocate on behalf of TGD people and ensure that the world is a safe place where TGD people "benefit from access to evidence-based health care, social services, justice, and equality."[12] Mental health providers who desire to work with TGD people should be aware that being prepared to provide advocacy is considered a basic aspect of being a culturally competent provider.[12] For example, the Standards of Care (SOC) suggest that providers should be prepared to engage in policy development that protects the rights of TGD people.[12]

The SOC established several recommendations for providers. These tasks include assessment, treatment, and appropriate referral for transition-related care.[12] One of the assumptions that is often made by mental health providers is a requirement for

---

[b] Don't Ask Don't Tell was a regulation in the US military that allowed for the discharge of lesbian, gay, and bisexual people if they were open about their sexual orientation. Furthermore, this regulation included protection for lesbian, gay, and bisexual people if they did not disclose their sexual orientation; superiors were not allowed to ask, if the military personnel did not tell. This regulation did not include protection for TGD people.

a certain length of mental health treatment. There is no absolute requirement either to engage in mental health treatment or that any treatment be of a specified length.[12] Mental health providers are in the best position to break down this erroneous belief. Too often TGD people are incorrectly informed that they must engage in mental health treatment for as long as 2 years. In the meantime, TGD people are paying for unnecessary care and are delayed in making social or medical transitions. Mental health providers must work to dismantle this inaccurate assumption about the amount and types of counseling and psychotherapy that are required. In short, the WPATH SOC state that "psychotherapy is not an absolute requirement for hormone therapy and surgery."[12] Each of the tasks that are outlined by the SOC can be engaged in from a social justice perspective. For example, when conducting assessments or diagnosing clients, providers are encouraged to have open and honest conversations with their clients about the limitations of assessment and the possible need for gender dysphoria diagnosis. Furthermore, if a gender dysphoria diagnosis is not necessary for a client to receive services, a provider should not unnecessarily provide one (See Stephanie L. Budge and lore m. dickey's article, "Barriers, Challenges, and Decision-Making in the Letter Writing Process for Gender Transition," in this issue).

Another important aspect of work with TGD clients is that counseling and psychotherapy are "not intended to alter a person's gender identity."[12] Rather, the intention of therapy and counseling is to ensure that the client has the skills necessary to cope with the day-to-day challenges they may face. Efforts to change, or alter, a person's gender identity fall into the category of reparative therapy. This type of treatment has been determined to be harmful for clients. Gender diversity is a natural human condition and there is no need to "correct" these people by expecting that they will conform to gender roles that are consistent with the sex they were assigned at birth.[11,17,18]

The SOC specifically call for mental health providers to advocate on behalf of their clients.[12] This might include working with a client's employer, school administrator, or health care provider to ensure that the client's needs in each of these settings are being met.[2,11] One of the ways that mental health providers can advocate for their clients is to write letters of referral or support for changes to identity documents (eg, birth certificate, driver's license, passport). Letter writing is an important part of the mental health provider's work with TGD clients. Readers should become familiar with the various aspects of what should be included in letters and what information is not necessary (eg, diagnostic impressions) (See Stephanie L. Budge and lore m. dickey's article, "Barriers, Challenges, and Decision-Making in the Letter Writing Process for Gender Transition," in this issue).[19]

### American Psychological Association

The American Psychological Association adopted as policy the Guidelines for Psychological Practice with Transgender and Gender Nonconforming People (hereafter referred to as "guidelines") in August of 2015.[11] There are 16 guidelines that cover a variety of applications in addition to concerns across the lifespan. These guidelines begin with foundational information that is considered to be the most basic information that mental health providers must have as they aspire to become culturally competent, trans-affirmative providers. Trans-affirmative care has been defined as "culturally-relevant for TGNC [transgender and gender nonconforming] clients and their multiple social identities, addresses the influence of social inequities on the lives of TGNC clients, enhances TGNC client resilience and coping, advocates to reduce systemic barriers to TGNC mental and physical health, and leverages TGNC client strengths."[20] To work from a culturally relevant perspective a provider must be aware of the differences between gender identity and sexual orientation and the ways in which these concepts inform one another.[11] Equally important is the need to have a strong understanding of the ways that multiple and marginalized identities can influence a TGD person's sense of well-being. For instance, trans people of color are at elevated risk of being victims of violence.[21] Finally, mental health providers are encouraged to explore their own sense of gender and the ways in which their identity may lead to unseen privilege that may complicate the development of rapport with clients (See lore m. dickey and colleagues' article, "Treatment of Trauma and Nonsuicidal Self-injury in Transgender Adults," in this issue).[11] For example, a cisgender provider may not be personally aware of the ways that TGD people struggle to deal with systemic barriers. When these issues become a part of the clinical discussion, cisgender people must evaluate their own assumptions about these challenges and refrain from minimizing the client's concerns.

The second domain covered by the guidelines addresses stigma, discrimination, and barriers to care. In this section, the ways in which TGD people are subject to violence and discrimination is discussed. These traumatic experiences can lead to complicated clinical concerns. For example, a TGD person may have come to therapy to address anxiety that seems to be the result of concerns in the client's workplace. As the clinical work deepens, it may become clear that some of the anxiety is the result of trauma the client has experienced. Mental health providers are encouraged to conduct a thorough assessment of trauma in a TGD person's life with the goal being to mitigate the consequences of these experiences (See lore m. dickey and colleagues' article, "Treatment of Trauma and Nonsuicidal Self-injury in Transgender Adults," in this issue).[22] Institutional barriers, including policies that reify the gender binary, have the potential to significantly impact a TGD person's life. The reasons for this include the myriad ways that such policies effectively erase the presence of TGD people in the public discourse. For example, if a person is unable to access medical care because of exclusionary language in their health insurance policy, it is possible that they will delay necessary health care. As a result, the emotional implications can be quite significant. This section ends with the need for mental health providers to understand their role in promoting "social change that reduces the negative effects of stigma."[11] Some mental health providers may balk at this expectation because they do not see this as an integral part of their work. However, as stated in the SOC, advocacy is considered to be a vital role for providers.[12]

The third domain covers lifespan considerations. In this section the guidelines address the needs of children and adolescents and older adults. The guideline that focuses on children and adolescents presents three approaches to working with children (eg, behavioral, affirmative, and wait-and-see approaches).[11] There is no consensus in the field about which approach has the best clinical outcome. Recent developments have discredited behavioral approaches to working with TGD children.[15] In behavioral approaches, gender-diverse youth are expected to learn to enjoy activities that conform with the expected gender roles that are consistent with the sex they were assigned at birth. These approaches have been shown to be harmful.[23] Affirmative approaches include either a wait-and-see approach or full support of a social transition.[17,18] Approaches to work with adolescents include the use of puberty blockers (eg, gonadotropin-releasing hormone treatment).[11,17,18] Puberty blockers are an effective way to address the psychological distress that is often associated with changes that occur as a result of puberty. This medical intervention suspends the effects of puberty and is completely reversible in that if a person stops taking the medication they will resume puberty. Supporting children and adolescents in affirming their gender identity has been shown to be predictive of positive outcomes.[24]

The final area in the lifespan section addresses work with TGD older adults. The needs of older adults have been largely overlooked in the literature. In this guideline, the needs of older adults are addressed including the challenges that some TGD people face when making a decision to transition later in life. In some cases, the decision to transition later in life is seen as being ambivalent about one's identity. The implication is that if a person waited until older adulthood to transition, then they are not clear about their identity.[11] There are many reasons why a person might wait until older adulthood to transition including family and work concerns.[25,26]

The fourth area of the guidelines addresses assessment, therapy, and interventions. This section covers topics including addressing co-occurring mental health concerns, the importance of social and clinical support, the ways in which transition may impact romantic relationships, the importance of addressing family creation, and the use of interdisciplinary teams to address the needs of clients. With regard to co-occurring clinical concerns, it is important to keep in mind that some TGD clients have clinical concerns that warrant attention. However it should not be assumed that the presence of these concerns precludes readiness for transition.[11,20] TGD people have healthy and loving romantic relationships.[11] Although historically TGD people were encouraged, if not required, to end relationships this is no longer the case. Some TGD people desire to create a family. It is important to discuss the implications of medical interventions (eg, hormones, puberty blockers) with clients because these interventions may impact the ability of a TGD person to provide genetic material (eg, eggs, sperm) for the purpose of creating a family.[27] One of the challenges when discussing this with adolescents is that they may not be prepared to make a decision about their desire to create a family at this developmental stage.[11,27]

The final guideline in this section addresses the importance of developing collaborative and interdisciplinary approaches to work with clients.[11,28] Although this is challenging for providers who are in rural or other underserved areas, it is still important to develop a strong group of providers across disciplines (eg, psychiatry, endocrinology, surgical, legal). This allows providers to have ready access to necessary referrals with providers with whom a collaborative relationship exists.[28]

The final domain of the guidelines addresses the areas of research, education, and training. In these guidelines the focus is on the importance of conducting research that supports knowledge of TGD people's lives without pathologizing their experiences. In the areas of education and training the guidelines address the importance of being competent to provide clinical services to TGD clients.[11] Little to no training is provided in most graduate training programs.[11] Although this is beginning to change, much still needs to be done to address the lack of training.

### American Counseling Association

The ACA counseling competencies for working with transgender clients have eight broad competency domains. Within each of these domains, there are individual competencies that detail how counselors should be working with trans clients. These competencies are training competencies, so the eight domains are helpful for all mental health professionals in terms of identifying how to work with trainees in these domains, and what the specific aspects of trans-affirmative counseling "look like" in actual practice. In using the ACA competencies, a provider is making a clear commitment to practice that includes an emphasis on social justice and advocacy.

The first domain, human growth and development, sets the stage for affirmative practice by acknowledging that trans people are an important part of the human spectrum of gender expression. Competency A.1 demonstrates this: Affirm that all persons have the potential to live full functioning and emotionally healthy lives throughout their mßäpäñ wflilu ürnDräüiny ma rüli äpäälrüm ül yänüär rläüuy äüpläälün, yänüär prä= sentation, and gender diversity beyond the male-female binary."[10]

The second domain, social and cultural foundations, describes the social context that transgender clients live within, and the importance of their multiple identities. For instance, competency B.5 asserts: "Recognize, acknowledge, and understand the intersecting identities of transgender people (eg, race/ethnicity, ability, class, religion/spiritual affiliation, age, experiences of trauma) and their accompanying developmental tasks. This should include attention to the formation and integration of the multiple identity statuses of transgender people."[10] Therefore, mental health practitioners are encouraged to view transgender people within not only the context of society, but also not assume that gender is the only focus of provider care.

The third domain, helping relationships, focuses on how rapport-building and trust are developed within the therapeutic relationship. Competency C.2 encourages mental health practitioners to "Recognize that the counselors' gender identity, expression, and concepts about gender are relevant to the helping relationship, and these identities and concepts influence the counseling process and may affect the counselor/client relationship.[10]

Within the fourth domain of group work, attention is provided to group modalities and how transgender clients may experience group work. For example, transgender clients will be alongside other cisgender members, and may experience the same type of discrimination and lack of information from their group peers as exemplified by D.1: "Maintain a nonjudgmental, supportive stance on all expressions of gender identity and sexuality and establish this as a standard for group members as well."[10]

The fifth domain, professional orientation, details the role of mental health practitioners not only within individual sessions, but extends the role of mental health practitioners to include advocacy within counseling settings at multiple levels. Competency E.9 reflects these multiple levels of mental health practitioner intervention through providing trans-affirmative information, and advocating with others when trans-negative and uninformed perspectives are noticed: "Recognize the importance of educating professionals, students, and supervisees about transgender issues, and challenge misinformation and bias about transgender individuals."[10]

For the sixth domain, career and lifestyle development, mental health practitioner advocacy includes an acknowledgment of the limitations of various assessments in career that are commonly used. These issues become critical when working with transgender clients, because there is tremendous employment discrimination that exists, so competency F.3 reminds mental health professionals to: "Acknowledge the potential problems associated with career assessment instruments that have not been normed for the transgender community."[10]

The seventh domain, appraisal, further attends to the domains of counseling and psychological assessment. The competencies within this domain revisit the therapeutic relationship and the role of advocacy in naming and challenging the gatekeeping role that mental health practitioners are placed within in transgender mental health care. Competency G.4 reads: "Examine the legitimate power that counselors hold as helping professionals, particularly in regards to assessment for body modifications, and seek to share information on the counselor's gate keeping role (eg, writing letters supporting body modifications) so it is not a restrictive influence, but rather seeks to better serve transgender people's needs."[10]

Finally, in the eighth domain of research, the competencies assert the importance of researchers exploring resilience and strength-based approaches to trans-affirmative care and scholarship, as reflected in competency H.1: "Be aware of existing transgender research and literature regarding social and emotional wellbeing and difficulties, identity formation, resilience and coping with oppression, as well as medical and non-medical treatment options."[10] The ACA competencies are a critical training document that can easily be incorporated into educational programs to help address the gap regarding clinical work with TGD people.

### American Psychiatric Association

The American Psychiatric Association's Position Statement on Access to Care for Transgender and Gender Variant Individuals[29] has helped move the field away from pathologizing gender identity. Although there are not formal competencies, guidelines, or standards within the American Psychiatric Association for trans-affirmative care, there has been movement away from a pathologic approach to working with transgender people. There has been a long-time pathologizing approach to care from the perspective of many mental health practitioners and transgender advocates, as evidenced by the restrictive diagnostic history within the *Diagnostic and Statistical Manual of Mental Disorders*[30] and the extensive gatekeeping psychiatrists have provided.

In 2012, the American Psychiatric Association issued a Position Statement on Access to Care for Transgender and Gender Variant Individuals,[29] which was grounded in four major values within the organization. One of these values includes patient advocacy: (1) best standards of clinical practice, (2) patient-focused treatment decisions, (3) scientifically established principles of treatment, and (4) advocacy for patient.

Within this position statement asserting the need for transgender people to have increased access to transgender-related medical care, the association proposed three major points that embed advocacy within the role of psychiatric treatment when working with transgender clients: (1) recognizes that appropriately evaluated transgender and gender-variant individuals can benefit greatly from medical and surgical gender transition treatments; (2) advocates for removal of barriers to care and supports public and private health insurance coverage for gender transition treatment; and, (3) opposes categorical exclusions of coverage for such medically necessary treatment when prescribed by a physician.[29]

This statement provided a tool for psychiatrists and other mental health practitioners to advocate with insurance companies and medical providers to initiate and increase transgender access to needed medical care. Psychiatrists may be closely involved with TGD people in caring for medical concerns. Having a strong understanding of the position taken by the American Psychiatric Association helps to ensure that clients receive affirming care.

## ADVOCACY RECOMMENDATIONS

There are four areas that merit attention with regard to recommendations for involvement in advocacy: (1) insurance coverage, (2) provider training, (3) structural practicalities, and (4) advocacy competencies.

### Insurance Coverage

There are two main issues with insurance coverage. The first is having access to coverage for basic medical care. Many people rely on their employer to provide health insurance; however, large numbers of TGD are unemployed or underemployed.[4] Although there have been recent changes in the insurance arena, universal coverage is far from the reality, and as a result many TGD people have trouble accessing affordable care.

The second concern regarding insurance coverage relates to the challenges people have in finding providers who are competent to provide care and accept the type of incur and is held by a TGD person. This is especially challenging for individuals who are covered by Medicare or Medicaid. It is not impossible to find a provider; however, there may be a need to travel great distances to find competent care.

### Provider Training

Far too often providers receive little to no training in how to work with gender-diverse people. Given that the field is rapidly changing it is critical that providers stay current in their knowledge of TGD people's lived experiences.[11] Training should include an understanding of identity development models (eg, exploring the ways in which a client develops their gender identity), consultation practice, supervision, knowledge of co-occurring mental health concerns (eg, depression, anxiety substance abuse), and how to work with interdisciplinary teams.

### Structural Practicalities

Structural practicalities refer to the ability of TGD people to work through the various challenges they may face. This includes having the ability to find resources, to advocate for one's needs, and to face the challenges that are often related to accessing care when one is TGD. For example, the first author needed to receive care for a chronic pain condition from a local emergency department. However, the provider was more interested in learning about how to work with TGD patients than she was in providing the care needed to address the pain. This experience of needing to educate one's provider is an inappropriate expectation on behalf of the provider. Clients should not be placed in the position where they are the educator.

### Advocacy Competencies

For some people, engaging in advocacy is an easy role; for others, it does not come naturally. Lewis and colleagues[31] have developed a framework for understanding advocacy in a mental health clinical setting. The domains identified in this model are:

a. Client empowerment
b. Client advocacy
c. Community collaboration
d. Systems advocacy
e. Public information
f. Social/political advocacy

In these domains the types of activities in which a provider might engage include developing self-advocacy for clients; helping clients to gain access to needed services; understand and acknowledge the client's resilience; and developing allies, including elected officials, with whom to partner for social and political change.[30]

### SUMMARY

Mental health providers are in an ideal position to engage in advocacy on behalf of TGD people. Historically, the field has had a turbulent history with TGD people. This problem is changing as providers adopt a trans-affirmative approach to their work. Understanding the ways that TGD people are adversely impacted by life stressors is an important first step in helping clients to overcome these challenges. Providers are encouraged to make a commitment to adopting a social justice perspective to their work with TGD clients and to make this approach known to those with whom they work.

## REFERENCES

1. Singh AA, Burnes TR. Shifting the counselor role from gate keeping to advocacy: ten strategies for using the ACA Competencies for Counseling with transgender clients into counseling, practice, research, and advocacy. J LGBT Issues Couns 2010;4:126–34.
2. dickey lm, Singh AA, Chang S, et al. Advocacy and social justice: the next generation of counseling and psychological practice with transgender and gender nonconforming clients. In: Singh AA, dickey lm, editors. Affirming counseling and psychological practice with transgender and gender nonconforming clients. Washington, DC: American Psychological Association; 2017. p. 247–62.
3. dickey lm, Budge SL, Katz-Wise SL, et al. Health disparities in the transgender community: exploring differences in insurance coverage. Psychol Sex Orientat Gend Divers 2016;3:275–82.
4. Grant JM, Mottet LA, Tanis J, et al. Injustice at every turn: a report of the national transgender discrimination survey. Washington, DC: National Center for Transgender Equality & National Gay and Lesbian Task Force; 2011. Available at: http://endtransdiscrimination.org/PDFs/NTDS_Report.pdf. Accessed July 28, 2016.
5. Institute of Medicine. The health of lesbian, gay, bisexual, and transgender people: building a foundation for better understanding. Washington, DC: National Academy of Sciences; 2011.
6. National Coalition of Anti-Violence Programs. Hate violence against lesbian, gay, bisexual, transgender, queer, and HIV-affected communities in the United States in 2011: a report from the National Coalition of Anti-Violence Programs. New York: Author; 2011. Available at: http://avp.org/storage/documents/Reports/2012_NCAVP_2011_HV_Report.pdf. Accessed July 28, 2016.
7. Goldblum P, Testa RJ, Pflum S, et al. In-school gender-based victimization and suicide attempts in transgender individuals. Prof Psychol Res Pr 2012;43:468–75.
8. Nuttbrock L, Bockting W, Rosenblum A, et al. Gender abuse and major depression among transgender women: a prospective study of vulnerability. Am J Public Health 2014;104(11):2191–8.
9. Center for Substance Abuse Treatment. A provider's introduction to substance abuse treatment for lesbian, gay, bisexual and transgender individuals (DHHS Pub. No. [SMA] 21-4104). Rockville (MD): U.S. Department of health and Human Services, Substance Abuse and Mental Health Services Administration, Center for Substance Abuse Treatment; 2012.
10. American Counseling Association. American Counseling Association competencies for counseling with transgender clients. J LGBT Issues Couns 2010;4:135–59.
11. American Psychological Association. Guidelines for psychological practice with transgender and gender nonconforming people. Am Psychol 2015;70(9):832–64.
12. Coleman E, Bockting W, Botzer M, et al. Standards of care for the health of transsexual, transgender, and gender nonconforming people, 7th version. Int J Transgend 2012;13:165–232.
13. Lewis JA, Ratts MV, Paladino DA, et al. Social justice counseling and advocacy: developing new leadership roles and competencies. J Soc Action Coun Psychol 2011;3:5–16.
14. Keisling M. Toward open military service. Available at: http://www.transequality.org/blog/toward-open-military-service. Accessed July 23, 2016.

15. Tobin HJ. Pentagon lifts transgender military service ban. Available at: http://www.transequality.org/blog/pentagon-lifts-transgender-military-service-ban. Accessed July 23, 2016.

16. Lev AI. Transgender emergence: therapeutic guidelines for working with gender-variant people and their families. New York: Haworth Clinical Press; 2004.

17. Edwards-Leeper L. Affirmative care of TGNC children and adolescents. In: Singh AA, dickey lm, editors. Affirming counseling and psychological practice with transgender and gender nonconforming clients. Washington, DC: American Psychological Association; 2017. p. 119–41.

18. Edwards-Leeper L, Leibowitz S, Sangganjanavanich VF. Affirmative care with transgender and gender nonconforming youth: expanding the model. Psychol Sex Orientat Gend Divers 2016;3(2):165–72.

19. Budge SL. Psychotherapists as gatekeepers: an evidence-based case study highlighting the role and process of letter writing for transgender clients. Psychotherapy (Chic) 2015;52(3):287–97.

20. Singh AA, dickey lm. Introduction. In: Singh AA, dickey lm, editors. Affirming counseling and psychological practice with transgender and gender nonconforming clients. Washington, DC: American Psychological Association; 2017. p. 3–18.

21. Singh AA, Hwahng SJ, Chang SC, et al. Affirmative counseling with trans/gender-variant people of color. In: Singh AA, dickey lm, editors. Affirming counseling and psychological practice with transgender and gender nonconforming clients. Washington, DC: American Psychological Association; 2017. p. 41–68.

22. Richmond K, Burnes TR, Singh AA, et al. Assessment and treatment of trauma with TGNC clients: a feminist approach. In: Singh AA, dickey lm, editors. Affirming counseling and psychological practice with transgender and gender nonconforming clients. Washington, DC: American Psychological Association; 2017. p. 191–212.

23. Substance Abuse Mental Health Services Administration. Ending conversion therapy: supporting and affirming LGBTQ youth. Rockville (MD): SAMHSA; 2016.

24. Olson KR, Durwood L, DeMeules M, et al. Mental health of transgender children who are supported in their identities. Pediatrics 2015;137(3):e20153223.

25. dickey lm, Bowers KL. Aging and TGNC identities: working with older adults. In: Singh AA, dickey lm, editors. Affirming counseling and psychological practice with transgender and gender nonconforming clients. Washington, DC: American Psychological Association; 2017. p. 161–74.

26. Porter KE, Brennan-Ing M, Chang S, et al. Providing competent and affirming services for transgender and gender nonconforming older adults. Clin Gerontol 2016; 39(5):366–88.

27. dickey lm, Ducheny KM, Ehrbar RD. Family creation options for transgender and gender nonconforming people. Psychol Sex Orientat Gend Divers 2016;3(2): 173–9.

28. Ducheny K, Hendricks ML, Keo-Meier C. TGNC-affirmative interdisciplinary collaborative care. In: Singh AA, dickey lm, editors. Affirming counseling and psychological practice with transgender and gender nonconforming clients. Washington, DC: American Psychological Association; 2017. p. 69–94.

29. American Psychiatric Association. Position statement on access to care for transgender and gender variant individuals. 2012. Available at: http://www.psychiatry.org/File%20Library/About-APA/Organization-Documents-Policies/Policies/Position-2012-Transgender-Gender-Variant-Access-Care.pdf?_ga=1.3365301.403197919.1469704033. Accessed July 28, 2016.

30. American Psychiatric Association. Diagnostic and statistical manual of mental disorders. 5th edition. Washington, DC: American Psychiatric Association; 2013.
31. Lewis, Arnold, House, et al. Advocacy competency domains. 2003. Available at: https://www.counseling.org/Resources/Competencies/Advocacy_Competencies. pdf. Accessed July 28, 2016.

# Past and Future Challenges Associated with Standards of Care for Gender Transitioning Clients

Lin Fraser, EdD[a],*, Gail Knudson, MD, MEd, FRCPC[b]

## KEYWORDS

- Standards of care • SOC 7 • World Professional Association for Transgender Health
- Gender dysphoria • Transsexual • Transgender • Gender nonconforming

## KEY POINTS

- WPATH has published seven versions (1979, 1980, 1981, 1990, 1998, 2001, and 2012) of Standards of Care (SOC), guidelines to provide safe and effective pathways for the health of transsexual, transgender, and gender nonconforming people. The general goal of psychotherapeutic, endocrine, or surgical therapy for gender transitioning clients is lasting personal comfort with their gendered selves to maximize overall psychological well-being and self-fulfillment.
- The main challenges associated with Standards of Care for gender transitioning clients are to stay current with the evolving evidence-base and evolving models of clinical practice, to be adaptable and culturally competent globally, and to be useful not only for practitioners but also other interested parties.
- The SOC are updated regularly and version 8 is in progress.

## INTRODUCTION

The World Professional Association for Transgender Health (WPATH) has produced seven versions of the Standards of Care (SOC) starting in 1979. Subsequent versions were published in 1980, 1981, 1990, 1998, 2001, and 2012. The SOC, also known as the Standards, are global guidelines to promote the health of transsexual, transgender, and gender nonconforming people and are used by providers, insurers, government bodies, and other stakeholders including consumers.

The authors have nothing to disclose.

[a] Private Practice, 2538 California Street, San Francisco, CA 94115, USA; [b] Faculty of Medicine, University of British Columbia, #201, 1770 Fort Street, Victoria, British Columbia V8R 1J5, Canada
* Corresponding author.
E-mail address: linfraser@gmail.com

Psychiatr Clin N Am 40 (2017) 15–27
http://dx.doi.org/10.1016/j.psc.2016.10.012
0193-953X/17/© 2016 Elsevier Inc. All rights reserved.

Their development and use had not been without challenges. These have been external and internal; externally to keep up with the changing content of evidence-based medicine consistent with the human rights of clients, and internally to meet the challenges of adaptable ethical use in practice. Because this article is written primarily for mental health professionals, the emphasis is to give clinicians context for understanding why the SOC have been written in the first place, their evolution over time, and on those challenges of most importance to this group in practice.

This article defines a standard of care, describes their purpose in general, and then moves into an overview of the WPATH SOC. Past challenges in general and those specifically connected to mental health are described. Then the current general process and challenges therein in developing SOC 7 followed by specific challenges for mental health professionals using them in practice are explored. The article concludes by reviewing challenges moving forward into the eighth version.

## WHAT ARE THE STANDARDS OF CARE?

A standard of care is a diagnostic and treatment process that a clinician should follow for a certain type of patient, illness, or clinical circumstance. In legal terms, it determines the level at which the average, prudent provider in a given community would practice. It is how similarly qualified practitioners would have managed the patient's care under the same or similar circumstances. In a legal proceeding, the medical malpractice plaintiff must establish the appropriate standard of care and demonstrate that the standard of care has been breached.[1]

Because a standard of care establishes a common protocol that an average, prudent provider should follow in a given setting, it provides a framework that is used for legal purposes advocating on behalf of the patient. A standard of care also promotes the use of a common language. A standard of care has an aim to ensure that clients or patients receive adequate and appropriate assessment, care, and treatment of their condition. Finally, and probably most importantly, a standard of care protects the public from substandard and dangerous medical practices.[2]

Formed in 1979, WPATH is the oldest and only global professional organization solely devoted to transgender health. WPATH is an international, multidisciplinary, professional association whose mission is to promote evidence-based care, education, research, advocacy, public policy, and respect in transgender health. The vision of WPATH is to bring together diverse professionals dedicated to developing best practices and supportive policies worldwide that promote health, research, education, respect, dignity, and equality for transsexual, transgender, and gender nonconforming people in all cultural settings.[3]

WPATH has produced the SOC outlining the best treatment protocols for transsexual, transgender, and gender nonconforming people wanting to pursue medical transition since 1979. There have been seven versions of this document with the most recent being published in 2012.[3–5] The overall goal of the SOC is to provide clinical guidance for health professionals to assist transsexual, transgender, and gender nonconforming people with safe and effective pathways to achieving lasting personal comfort with their gendered selves, to maximize their overall health, psychological well-being, and self-fulfillment.[3] Although the SOC recognize that language is evolving and numerous terms are used to describe one's gender identity, three terms (transsexual, transgender, and gender nonconforming) are used consistently throughout the document to maximize the number of identities included. The guidelines are based on expert medical consensus and where possible, evidence-based medicine. Although the SOC aim to be global, the authors recognize that some of its applicability may be limited in developing nations and therefore the clinical guidelines must be flexible and adaptable.

The guidelines have evolved over time according to the cultural climate of Western Europe and North America. The first versions of the SOC were based on a prescriptive sex change model. People wanting gender-affirming surgery were required to follow a set of steps to be eligible for surgery. The early documents ranged from 7 to 10 pages, were based on professional consensus, and contained no references. The most recent version is 111 pages and includes more than 100 references. This current version, although the most evidence-based to date, is still based partially on clinical consensus, and focuses not only on medical transition, but on the overall health care of transsexual, transgender, and gender nonconforming people.[6]

## CHALLENGES WITH THE STANDARDS OF CARE OVER TIME
### General Challenges

In 1979, a follow-up study of the people who had surgery at the Johns Hopkins Clinic reported no difference or a decreased quality of life, which led to closure of the clinic.[7,8] Shortly thereafter, with the prospect of the closure of other gender identity clinics, a small group of health care professionals who were determined to continue medical treatment of their transsexual patients began the process of developing a standard of care to determine eligibility for what was then called sex reassignment surgery. This then led to the first SOC authored by Johns Hopkins–trained medical psychologist Paul Walker, PhD and his team. These were approved in 1979 by the attendees of one of the first symposia of the newly formed Harry Benjamin International Gender Dysphoria Association (HBIGDA), later to become WPATH. Another event led to the formation of the first SOC: surgery on demand in a garage in San Francisco. The original SOC was produced to protect clients seeking medical transition and to protect the reputation of health care professionals involved in this field.[4,9]

### Challenge in Providing Care Without Professional Support or Nomenclature

In the early years, gender normative views of transgender people portrayed them as suffering from serious pathology and a mental disorder that could only be treated by mental health professionals. However, HBIGDA believed in a combination of psychological and medical treatment to improve the quality of life for their patients. One challenge was to create a document that could include medical interventions known as the triadic sequence, a year of living in the gender role consistent with their self-concept, known then as the "life-test," along with cross-sex hormones and sex-reassignment surgery. The biggest challenges came from within the medical community because the early SOC were created with little support from even other professionals in the small field of transgender health. These pioneering professionals risked professional ostracism to ensure quality care for their patients. There was no nomenclature for the condition in the Diagnostic and Statistical Manual of Mental Disorders (DSM); the closest diagnosis at the time was transvestism, which fell under the parent sexual deviations in DSM-II. The International Classification of Diseases (then ICD-9) did, however, include the diagnosis of transvestism and transsexualism under the parent of sexual deviation. The subsequent DSM (DSM-III) published in 1980 introduced the diagnoses of transsexualism under the parent of Psychosexual Disorders.[9] The early pioneers in HBIGDA referred to the condition as gender dysphoria and transsexualism interchangeably. The term transgender did not exist, coming into favor via the community as first a middle ground term between transsexual and transvestite, and then by 1994 as an umbrella term for all trans identities.[9]

In the early years there was no evidence base, no Internet, only a small group of health care professionals who believed that medical interventions helped, based on listening to their clients' narratives The accepted science of the day was an understanding of gender/sex based on a binary model of male/man and female/woman and clients also described themselves in those terms. Treatment involved providing medical interventions to move from one sex to the other.[9] The SOC described eligibility and readiness criteria for hormones and surgery. For example, people needed to be in psychotherapy for 3 months before starting hormones and 6 months before they would be eligible for surgery as long as they had been also cross-living for at least a year. Although these criteria were later seen as barriers to care, at the time, there would have been no medical treatment without them. Hence, clients were extremely appreciative that health care professionals involved in this small field developed standards by which they could receive gender-affirming surgery and also legitimize their experience.

### Challenges with the Changing Evidence-Base

It is beyond the scope of this article to describe the challenges faced during the periods of intervening versions of the SOC up to the present day, but a description of the early history can give the reader context for the remainder of the article. Although the types of challenges faced by the original authors were more extensive than faced today, each subsequent version of the SOC was developed to be able to ensure up-to-date ethical, competent, and compassionate care to their clients and each faced its own challenges.

Times have changed dramatically from the early days, as has the gradual scientific understanding that gender is not binary, but exists on a spectrum.[3] Although Harry Benjamin recognized this gender diversity in the 1960s, this understanding did not emerge in the SOC until SOC 7.[3,10] The reader is referred to the section about advancements in the knowledge and treatment of gender dysphoria in SOC 7 for further information.[3] The literature indicates that the use of hormones and surgery is effective for many people but that everyone seeking care does not fit within the binary model of gender. SOC 7 mentions that treatments should be individualized and tailored to the needs of a diverse population.[3] Thus, the SOC has changed as a result of increased knowledge and a growing evidence-base. For example, even by the time that SOC 5 was published in 1998, many transgender people were finding ways to comfortably express themselves that did not follow the original "triadic sequence" of therapy.[11]

### Challenge in Balancing Ethical Practice with Human Rights

As time has passed, trans people themselves have been able to take a more active role in the development of the SOC with the rise of the Internet allowing the development of activist and knowledgeable communities requesting changes to the SOC based on their lived experiences. For example, for SOC 7, an international advisory committee of community members was formed that commented on the successive drafts of the current version, allowing a give and take between members of the writing committee and representatives of the community.[3] The outcome of such ongoing conversations seems to have been beneficial to all parties. There had been tensions between leaders from the community requesting fewer barriers to care and more personal autonomy, with those providers given the responsibility of developing ethical medical guidelines. The issue still remains to balance ethical practice with human rights regarding autonomy related to one's own body. But as time has passed, there is less separation between providers and trans clients. Many trans people have

---

**Box 1**
**WPATH de-psychopathologization statement – May 26, 2010**

The WPATH Board of Directors strongly urges the de-psychopathologization of gender variance worldwide. The expression of gender characteristics, including identities, that are not stereotypically associated with one's assigned sex at birth is a common and culturally-diverse human phenomenon which should not be judged as inherently pathologic or negative. The psychopathologization of gender characteristics and identities reinforces or can prompt stigma, making prejudice and discrimination more likely, rendering transgender and transsexual people more vulnerable to social and legal marginalization and exclusion, and increasing risks to mental and physical well-being. WPATH urges governmental and medical professional organizations to review their policies and practices to eliminate stigma toward gender-variant people.

*From* The World Professional Association for Transgender Health, Inc. WPATH de-psychopathologization statement. May 26, 2010. Available at: http://www.wpath.org/site_page.cfm?pk_association_webpage_menu=1351&pk_association_webpage=3928. Accessed October 1, 2016; with permission.

---

become health care providers themselves and have joined the ranks of the SOC committee.

### Challenges with Changes in Nomenclature and Diagnoses

The field of research has grown exponentially since the 1970s; however, evidence-based medicine is still lacking in many areas. Changes in culture have also led to the gradual depathologization of transgender identities in Western Europe and North America. The way in which gender dysphoria is viewed has changed within the nomenclature consistent with this gradual depathologization. The SOC have followed suit and WPATH has even led the way (**Box 1**). For example, the diagnoses in the DSM changed from transsexualism (DMS-III, 1980) to Gender Identity Disorder (DSM- IV, 1994 and DSM-IV-TR, 2000) to Gender Dysphoria (DSM-5, 2013; and SOC 7).[9]

SOC 7 includes a definition of gender dysphoria that purports a nonbinary approach to gender identity, and notes that it is the distress of the dysphoria that can meet a formal diagnosis of a disorder rather than the person's gender identity itself being a disorder. Although DSM-5 was in draft form and was not released before the publication of SOC 7, WPATH had been asked to advise on the section related to gender identity diagnosis and suggested the name gender dysphoria, a much less pathologizing term than the former gender identity disorder.[9] The ICD revision was also in process and the diagnosis of transsexualism will most likely be changed to gender incongruence and moved into a new chapter on sexual health.[12] Language in the nomenclature of DSM, ICD, and the SOC is thus meant to be nonpathologizing of identities, while at the same time providing access to needed care. This gradual depathologization has resulted in reduced barriers to care and more flexibility in the SOC.

### Challenges with Models of Care

Nevertheless, it is generally understood that there is value in providing standards to guide health care, which would still include transgender health care. Rather than being a prescriptive document as seen in the earlier versions, SOC 7 is focused on promoting optimal overall health care of transsexual, transgender, and gender nonconforming people.

Some trans people may prefer an informed consent model rather than upselne stan dards they have to follow. As a flexible document, SOC 7 does not preclude using this type of model, particularly in multidisciplinary centers where mental health practitioners are easily available for referral and consultation. A major challenge still lies in determining eligibility to access medical transition when serious psychological concerns are not well controlled, and/or major social considerations or complications may exist, particularly related to children and adolescents. Ultimately, it is important to ensure that the SOC are trans affirmative and do not contribute adversely to problems with providers in a gate-keeping role.

The SOC are based on a medical model. For example, the first SOC required psychotherapy before cross-sex hormones prescription. Two referral letters were needed for surgery, both written by doctoral level mental health providers, at least one by a psychiatrist, and the other by a psychologist or psychiatrist.[13] These requirements gradually changed to one by doctoral level and the other by at least a Master's level clinician.[11,14] The SOC 7 has now further changed so that Master's level clinicians can write both letters. In addition, primary care physicians, nurses, and nurse practitioners that meet similar criteria as mental health practitioners (specialized training in behavioral diagnosis and assessment) can also do their own assessments for hormones. These changes came about to reduce barriers to care as more interdisciplinary providers became trained in trans health. There was also the growing evidence-base that supported recent professional consensus that gender nonconformity in and of itself was not a mental disorder. Authors of the DSM-5 were clear that the diagnosis was based on the distress caused by the dysphoria and not the trans person's gender identity itself.[15] By the time SOC 6 was published, psychotherapy was no longer a prerequisite, although it is still recommended especially in complex cases.[3,14] Moreover, informed consent is an emerging practice model in North America and is described briefly as a possible model for care in SOC 7. This is a departure from the classic mental health–based model.

Because of the move away from the binary model of gender identity as a prerequisite for medical transition, more gender diverse people are presenting for care.[16,17] The SOC promote more individualized care to include all identities but guidelines are sparse leaving the practitioner with little specific information about how to assist with nonbinary transitions. Moreover, increasing numbers of people experiencing financial, mental health, and social barriers are able to access care but also require more assistance in their social and medical transition than those experiencing fewer barriers. The mental health needs of these clients may be higher than previously seen clients and their situations may be more complex. As for nonbinary identities, the SOC offer little guidance for those with more complicated social needs, such as postoperative care for the homeless. Although the practitioner now has more flexibility and can tailor an individualized approach for each client, they may be left with a challenge of not having enough guidance to offer the best care given these increasingly complex cases coming to their practices.

### Challenges with Staying Flexible with Greater Global Diversity

The field is moving fast despite a general lack of evidence-based medicine. There has to be a capacity to respond to the demand for care within the current knowledge base and allow for what is not known. The SOC is based on a Western perspective and is challenging to adapt globally. Historically, it was based on a binary model of gender identity and this has changed with subsequent versions. The newer SOC acknowledge that trans people in non-Western cultures who come for care may have different needs than those in North America and Western Europe. People who identify as nonbinary or genderqueer are also seeking care and treatment globally.[17] The SOC does not describe a current understanding of gender identities across all cultures nor does it offer complete guidelines for nonbinary identities. Hence, it is not able to act as a universal guide for cultural competency. What it does instead is allow for flexibility and adaptation.

There is an ongoing challenge to respond to the needs of the various constituents. The SOC is written primarily for practitioners but is also used by insurance companies, governments, and the community. In this way the SOC has to be useful for law but broad enough that people can adapt to their local area or constituencies.

At this point WPATH is only beginning to train people in using the SOC, but with the advent of the Global Education Initiative it is hoped that this training will take place across the world.[4] Promoting and marketing the most recent versions of the SOC has also been a challenge. Although the newest versions are available for download free online at www.wpath.org, an Android or IOS application would be helpful. This would enable people to be aware of the current SOC rather than practicing the old ones, because updated versions would always be available.

The SOC is constantly evolving and has the challenge of meeting the needs of rapidly changing constituencies. This is difficult, because the clinician has the responsibility of knowing both the content of the SOC and principles of ethical practice. By the time the SOC are published, parts may be out of date with current practice and rapidly evolving research. It would be helpful to have online versions that could be quickly updated.

## CHALLENGES OF ACCESS TO CARE

When writing SOC 7, the SOC Committee determined the audience, set the tone, and developed the content. The current literature was reviewed and review papers written in the decided content areas. The most recent SOC is geared to focus on transgender health and how the health care professional can improve the lives of transsexual, transgender, and gender nonconforming people. This is different from prior versions that were more prescriptive and described detailed steps that transgender people had to follow to access health care.[3]

Another significant shift in the most recent version of the SOC is that gender identity is no longer seen as pathologic. The gender dysphoria experienced by people may be alleviated through social and or medical transition. However, some countries have accepted people living across genders and between genders as in integral part of their society without medical transition. Where possible, evidence-based medicine was used in preparing the content (eg, endocrine therapy and cancer-screening protocols). However, some of the recommendations remain based on professional consensus.

Another area of change is the inclusion of family practice physicians and nurses in hormonal and surgical care planning for people wishing to medically transition. It is hoped that this will more easily enable people to access care globally. Health care professionals residing mostly in Western Europe and North America where most of the research originates, wrote the current and past SOC guidelines. In the most recent version, an International Community Advisory Committee was established to review the content.

Although the SOC aims to be global, the authors recognize that some of its applicability may be limited in developing nations. In this way the inclusion of primary care professionals and possibly someday paraprofessionals may help in increasing access to care for those in the developing world. The current SOC also includes another way to increase access to care, and that is by including guidelines for telehealth. The use of

---
**BOX 2**
**International Advisory Committee feedback**

If I had to sum it up then it would be that whereas previous versions of the SOC were always perceived to be about the things that a trans person must do to satisfy clinicians, this version is much more clear about every aspect of what clinicians ought to do in order to properly serve their clients. That is a truly radical reversal, one that serves both parties very well. —Christine Burns.

---

e-therapy is a rapidly expanding area of mental health care and is especially helpful in rural or remote areas where access to gender-affirming health care may be lacking.[18] Assessment by videoconference is becoming more available. The clinician, however, must work within the guidelines and licensing laws of the jurisdiction.

SOC 7 also recognizes the role of informed consent and harm reduction approaches. For example, in recommending hormone therapy, the mental health professional must ensure that the client understands the psychological and physical benefits and risks of hormone therapy, and its psychosocial implications. In addition, the clinician must be able to diagnose gender dysphoria. This type of approach may also increase access to care. Nevertheless, SOC 7, in contrast to informed consent models, stresses the important role the mental health professional can play in the psychosocial adjustment for many transgender individuals throughout transition.[3]

Treatment of children and adolescents is becoming more commonplace and more accepted in several countries, although there is caution regarding irreversible medical interventions for minors. Children and adolescents are encouraged to explore their gender expression and health care professionals are advised to not impose a binary view of gender expression on their clients. Children who wish to explore social transition are allowed to do so within a safe environment and clinicians should approach the work in a balanced and affirmative manner.[19,20] When it comes to hormones and surgery, providers are encouraged to be especially mindful of balancing youth autonomy with ethical practice and specialists in child and adolescent health must be especially conscientious in the provision of affirmative and individualized care. For example, hormonal intervention is appropriate for some adolescents. Adolescents with gender dysphoria desiring masculinizing chest surgery are often approved providing they have met the criteria, including such factors as that there are no significant risks and they have good parental or caretaker/guardian involvement to support the treatment process.[3,19] Genital surgery is usually delayed until the person is older than the age of majority in a given country. There is a clear statement that withholding treatment is not a neutral option for adolescents because it "might prolong gender dysphoria and contribute to an appearance that could provoke abuse and stigmatization".[3] p.21 It should also be noted that reparative or conversion therapy is no longer considered ethical by the American Medical Association and the American Psychological Association.

Despite the challenges in the process of developing the current SOC, the public, community, and clinician response compared with past revisions has been close to universally positive.[5] The reader is referred to the comments in **Box 2** of International Advisory Board Member Christine Burn's statement for an elaboration of the general reception of SOC 7.

## CHALLENGES FOR MENTAL HEALTH PROFESSIONALS
### Dual Role as Assessor and Clinician

One big challenge for mental health professionals is around assessment. To write a comprehensive letter to support cross-sex hormone treatment and gender-affirming surgery, the clinician needs to build a therapeutic alliance with the client. The client may believe that they are there to "jump through hoops" and be reluctant to engage in the process. Moreover, the clinician may think that the client needs psychotherapy to ensure a successful medical transition. If the client disagrees, complex clinical situations may materialize.

The tasks related to assessment and referrals as written in the SOC 7 are as follows[3]:

1. Assess gender dysphoria
2. Goals of psychotherapy are broad and wide-ranging
3. Assess, diagnose, and discuss treatment options for coexisting mental health concerns
4. If applicable, assess eligibility, prepare, and refer for hormone therapy
5. If applicable, assess eligibility, prepare, and refer for surgery

The tasks related to psychotherapy in SOC 7 are very different:

1. Psychotherapy is not an absolute requirement for hormone therapy and surgery
2. Goals of psychotherapy for adults with gender concerns
3. Psychotherapy for transsexual, transgender, and gender nonconforming clients, including counseling and support for changes in gender role
4. Family therapy or support for family members
5. Follow-up care throughout life
6. E-therapy, online counseling, or distance counseling
7. Educate and advocate on behalf of clients within their community (schools, workplaces, other organizations) and assist clients with making changes in identity documents
8. Provide information and referral for peer support

There is a delicate balance between education of the client about the risks/benefits involved in medical transition versus a gatekeeping model. The dual role of assessor and therapist can foster a power imbalance between client and mental health professional, creating challenges to establishing rapport. Complex transference-countertransference situations may emerge especially if the clinical relationship is new. Even for those freely electing therapy, multiple sessions may be needed to establish trust, and a way to work together to reach the goals agreed on at the outset. This may be especially challenging for clients with a history of maltreatment in the health care system.[21,22] Navigating this dual relationship in a way that is ethical clinically and fair to the client can be problematic for both involved in this instance.

### Clinician Interpretation and Beliefs About Standards of Care

Because the SOC are written as a flexible document, clinicians have varying opinions about how to interpret its content. These differences may lead to miscommunications and expectations between the client and mental health professional. In addition, some clinicians may have personal beliefs that the SOC are too pathologizing and may be reluctant to ask questions related to their client's mental health (eg, depression, anxiety, substance use, autism spectrum, suicide ideation and attempts, history of trauma), and thus put the client at greater risk postoperatively because of the stress associated with major surgery. It is also important to note that studies involving co-occurring medical and mental health conditions with gender dysphoria have not been extrapolated on regarding how these may affect the perioperative period. For example, cigarette smoking adversely affects any kind of surgery outcome or if

~~line has a history of depression, a higher probability exists of having a postoperative~~ depression.[23]

### Gaps in Clinician Knowledge

There is also no guarantee mental health clinicians are cognizant of the risks and benefits of cross-sex hormone treatment and gender-affirming surgery or able to answer medical questions posed by the client. Most mental health professionals are not medically trained and yet often have more time with the client than do their medical providers. This may be one advantage for using an interdisciplinary team and communicating with their primary health care professional or endocrinologist in this area of the client's care planning because of their medical training. In cases where no mental health professionals are involved, will most primary care practitioners know when it is appropriate to refer to a mental health professional for consultation and second opinion? WPATH aims to resolve these dilemmas by providing interdisciplinary training for all health care providers. For example, The Global Education Initiative Foundations Courses provide licensed clinicians from multidisciplinary backgrounds with much needed, basic education regarding cultural competency, mental health, the use of cross-sex hormone treatment, gender-affirming surgeries, mental health and cultural competency, and the basics of assessment and medical transition planning.[4] Nonbinary gender identities were introduced in SOC 7 and a myriad of gender expressions (eg, agender) are becoming more prevalent.[16,17,24] These emerging gender identities are not mentioned in the current version and need to be included in the next version.

### Challenges Working with Children and Youth

The directive around youth gonadectomy and genital surgery is the age of majority in a given country. However, the age of majority does not necessarily correlate with health care decisions that youth are able to make without the consent of their parent and/or guardian. It is important to consider that no studies exist on the outcome of youth younger than the age of 18 having surgery and this is an important area for future research. In the meantime, an individualized, flexible, and careful approach is recommended.[20] Another area that is mentioned around children and adolescents is the notion of social transition of minors. At the time that the SOC 7 was written, few children were undergoing a social transition and this number has increased. The SOC 8 needs to include current research in this area, because few studies were available on the release of the document.

### CHALLENGES MOVING FORWARD
#### Informed Consent and Cultural Differences

There are several challenges related to moving forward with future development of the SOC. For one, the Standards need to become more descriptive of an informed consent model, at least for those providers who work within an interdisciplinary team or in areas where there are problems with access to care. Moreover, there may be, in many cases, a difference in health literacy with the health care provider being much more knowledgeable than the client. For example, what will be the outcome when the client disagrees with the opinion of the assessor? One must also consider cultural differences with respect to authority. For example, the client from a hierarchal culture may not feel comfortable with an informed consent model. Literature on cultural differences suggests that cultures labeled hierarchal have clear layers of social status. In these cultures, physicians have high social status and patients in these cultures might be socialized to expect the doctor to tell them what to do rather than making the decision more for themselves.[25]

## Letters and Criteria

In addition, fewer mental health professional referral letters with respect to gonadectomy are being proposed for SOC 8.[26] This could mean a mental health clinician not involved in psychotherapy may write the recommendation letter with the client. The second assessment might then be done by the urologist/gynecologist who is performing the gonadectomy.

With the criteria for age around surgery most likely declining, a question that emerges is this: what factors will be used to determine that the youth has capacity to consent for surgery? Chest surgery is a less invasive surgery than genital reconstructive surgeries and plastic surgery can be used to reconstruct the breasts if preferred so the risk is less if a person changes their mind later in life after having surgery. However, gonadectomy results in permanent loss of fertility and although options for fertility preservation must be discussed, these options may not be available because they are prohibitively expensive. What is unknown is whether the youth younger than 18 has the capacity to consent for gonadectomy without fertility preservation given that childbearing is not a common goal within that stage of development and the immaturity of the executive functioning of the brain. Also, it is difficult to predict whether they will wish to have children later in life. A second question is, does the youth have the capacity to consent for genital surgery, given the aforementioned reasons or the ability to appreciate the amount of aftercare needed postvaginoplasty and the number of surgeries and aftercare needed for phalloplasties? The opposing argument is that if the youth has the capacity for surgery and has good parental/guardian/caretaker support, their quality of life may improve (**Box 3**).

---

**Box 3**
**Challenges for clinicians**

- Multiple roles
  - Dual role as therapist and assessor
  - Tension between being an advocate and creating a "safe space" inside the consulting room
- Keeping abreast of evidence
- Continuing education in interdisciplinary fields, knowledge of other specialties
- Ethical practice and human rights

---

## SUMMARY

The biggest challenges and goals remain and always have been about reducing barriers and providing access to universal culturally competent compassionate health care for all transsexual, transgender, and gender nonconforming people (or whatever name a trans person might use as the language evolves). Yet much has changed. More expressions of gender identity are discussed in the current SOC, moving away from binary identities. The topic of transgender health has become more a mainstream topic in Western Europe and North America.[4] Transgender health has gained more respectability and the number of publications in academic journals is increasing. In addition, more multicenter trials are taking place, and research in evidence-based medicine. This respectability, strong evidence base, multiple identities, and

multicenter trials were hardly imaginable to the small group of pioneering professionals who developed the first SOC in 1979. SOC 8 promises to be even more inclusive, evidence-based, comprehensive, global, and culturally competent than any
previous versions. However, the view remains centered in the perspective of Western
Europe and North America and needs to become more globally focused.

There has also been an increase in the number of transgender health care providers
and more participatory action research projects have been published. Transgender
participation has increased and it seems that the community is less critical of the content of the current SOC. This may be because it is focused on health care and not as
prescriptive but there is also better communication among stakeholders. Nevertheless, there continues to be a tension between ethical practice and the human rights
perspective of autonomy, which can lead to a misunderstanding about the intentions
of the practitioner.

The field is moving so fast, it is difficult to keep abreast of the changes. Therefore,
one is always grappling with staying culturally competent to serve the community to
the best of their ability. Challenges will continue in this ever-evolving field but each
version has provided better guidelines for improved access, removal of barriers,
and better health care for trans people. There is hope that this positive evolution will
continue.

## REFERENCES

1. Richards EP, Rathbun KC. Medical care law. Gaithersburg (MD): As pen Publishers; 1999.
2. Annas GJ. Standard of care: the law of American Bioethics. New York: Oxford
   University Press; 1997.
3. Coleman E, Bockting W, Botzer M, et al. Standards of Care for the Health of Transsexual, Transgender, and Gender-Nonconforming People, Version 7. Int J Transgenderism 2012;13(4):165–232.
4. Wylie K, Knudson G, Khan SI, et al. Serving transgender people: clinical care
   considerations and service delivery models in transgender health. Lancet
   2016;388(10042):401–11.
5. Fraser L, Knudson G. Gender dysphoria and transgender health. In: Wylie K, editor. ABC of sexual health. West Sussex: Wiley Blackwell; 2015. p. 108–11.
6. Fraser L. Standards of care, transgender health. In: Whelehan P, Bolin A, editors.
   International Encyclopedia of Human Sexuality. Hoboken (NJ): Wiley-Blackwell
   Press; 2015.
7. Meyer JK, Reter D. Sex reassignment follow-up. Arch Gen Psychiatry 1979;36(9):
   1010–5.
8. Abramowitz SI. Psychosocial outcomes of sex reassignment surgery. J Consult
   Clin Psychol 1986;54(2):183–9.
9. Fraser L. Gender dysphoria: definition and evolution through the years. In:
   Trombetta C, editor. Management of gender dysphoria, a multidisciplinary
   approach. Milan (Italy): Springer; 2015. p. 19–31.
10. Benjamin H. The transsexual phenomenon. New York: Julian Press; 1966.
11. Levine SB, Brown GR, Coleman E, et al. The standards of care for gender identity
    disorders. J Psychol Human Sex 1998;11(2):1–34.
12. Drescher J, Cohen-Kettenis P, Winter S. Minding the body: situating gender iden-
    tity diagnoses in the ICD-11. Int Rev Psychiatry 2012;24(6):568–77.
13. Walker P, Berger J, Green R, et al. Standards of care. The hormonal and surgical
    sex-reassignment of gender dysphoric persons. 1979.

14. Meyer W, Bockting WO, Cohen-Kettenis P, et al. The Harry Benjamin International Gender Dysphoria Association's Standards of Care for Gender Identity Disorders, Sixth Version. J Psychol Human Sex 2002;13(1):1–30.
15. American Psychiatric Association. Diagnostic and statistical manual of mental disorders. 5th edition. Washington, DC: Author; 2013.
16. Chang SC, Rossman K. Gender and sexual orientation diversity within the TGNC community. In: Singh AA, editor. Affirmative counseling and psychological practice with transgender and gender nonconforming clients. Washington, DC: American Psychological Association; 2016. p. 19–40.
17. Richards C, Bouman WP, Seal L, et al. Non-binary or genderqueer genders. Int Rev Psychiatry 2016;28(1):95–102.
18. Fraser L. Etherapy: ethical and clinical considerations for version 7 of the World Professional Association for Transgender Health's Standards of Care. Int J Transgenderism 2009;11(4):247–63.
19. Edwards-Leeper L, Leibowitz S, Sangganjanavanich VF. Affirmative practice with transgender and gender nonconforming youth: expanding the model. Psychol Sex Orientat Gend Divers 2016;3(2):165–72.
20. Leibowitz S. Gender dysphoria and nonconformity and the pre-pubertal child, understanding clinical issues and gender development, mental health and hormonal treatment in adolescents. 2016.
21. Institute of Medicine. The health of lesbian, gay, bisexual, and transgender people: building a foundation for better understanding. Washington, DC: National Academy of Sciences; 2011.
22. Grant JM, Mottet LA, Tanis J, et al. Injustice at every turn: a report of the national transgender discrimination survey. Washington, DC: National Center for Transgender Equality & national gay and Lesbian task Force; 2011. Available at: http://endtransdiscrimination.org/pdfs/ntds_report.pdf.
23. Sørensen LT. Wound healing and infection in surgery. Ann Surg 2012;255(6):1069–79.
24. Van Caenegem EV, Wierckx K, Elaut E, et al. Prevalence of gender nonconformity in Flanders, Belgium. Arch Sex Behav 2015;44(5):1281–7.
25. Livermore D. Customs of the world: using cultural intelligence to adapt wherever you are, lecture 4: authority-low vs high power distance. Chantilly (VA): Great Courses; 2013.
26. Bouman W, Richards C, Addinall R, et al. Yes and yes again: are standards of care which require two referrals for genital reconstructive surgery ethical? Sex Relationship Ther 2014;29(4):377–89.

# Transgender and Gender Diverse Clients with Mental Disorders

## Treatment Issues and Challenges

Lauren Mizock, PhD

## KEYWORDS

- Transgender • Gender diversity • Mental health • Mental disorders • Treatment

## KEY POINTS

- Increased rates of suicidality, anxiety, and depression occur among transgender and gender diverse individuals.
- Gender variance can also impact the presentation of eating, psychotic, and autism spectrum disorders.
- Mental health disparities are largely impacted by transphobia and gender-related discrimination and abuse.
- Initial gender dysphoria may contribute to anxiety and distress, although this is often resolved with gender affirmation and gender-responsive care.

## INTRODUCTION

Transgender and gender diverse (TGD) individuals face risks of mental health problems and suicidality, often as a result of transphobia and minority stress. There are a number of resilience and protective factors that transgender individuals use to cope with mental health challenges and thrive. In this article, a review of the literature on the mental health risks faced by transgender individuals is provided, as well as a discussion of the protective factors that enhance resilience.

It is important to bring to this discussion an awareness of the tendency to pathologize the mental health of transgender individuals. Gender and sexual minority identities have been designated as mental illnesses in past editions of the *Diagnostic and*

Disclosure Statement: The author does not have a conflict of interest or direct financial interest in the subject matter or materials discussed in the article or with a company making a competing product.
Fielding Graduate University, Clinical Psychology PhD Program, 3610 Sacramento Street, San Francisco, CA 94118, USA
*E-mail address:* lmizock@fielding.edu

Psychiatr Clin N Am 40 (2017) 29–39
http://dx.doi.org/10.1016/j.psc.2016.10.008
0193-953X/17/© 2016 Elsevier Inc. All rights reserved.

**psych.theclinics.com**

*Statistical Manual of Mental Disorders* (DSM), including homosexuality, transsexualism, gender identity disorder, and other diagnoses. This history demonstrates the social construction of mental illness for lesbian, gay, bisexual, and transgender individuals in diagnoses that reflect dominant social and cultural norms for sexuality and gender.[1] Gender dysphoria and transvestic fetishism remain in the current DSM-5 as diagnoses, but not without some controversy.[2] In the present article, a discussion of mental health disparities is contextualized within a model of gender minority stress, and counterbalanced with a discussion of the resilience and coping that TGD individuals access to overcome these challenges.

## TRANSPHOBIA AND GENDER MINORITY STRESS

Transphobia, or stigma toward transgender identities, plays a key role in mental health disparities among gender diverse groups. Stigma can interfere with recovery from mental health problems and discrimination by reducing one's social status, social network, and self-esteem.[3] Transphobia often begins in childhood and adolescence, and includes such experiences as rejection by family and friends, insults from strangers, physical violence, or sexual assault.[4] Transgender people face both external stigma, which is prejudice and discrimination from others, as well as internalized transphobia, which is stigma that is taken on and directed at oneself. Both types of stigma can interfere with daily functioning and contribute to psychological distress and suicidality.[4–6]

The Gender Minority Stress Model[7] is an adaptation of the Minority Stress Model for lesbian, gay, and bisexual individuals,[8] and explains the increased rates of mental health problems among transgender individuals. The model delineates that stressful events, anticipatory stigma, and internalized transphobia can pose psychological distress and contribute to the onset of mental health problems.

Violent and nonviolent forms of discrimination can increase the risk of depression, anxiety, distress, and substance use.[9,10] Not passing may also present risk of discrimination and contribute to more psychological distress, depression, and suicide.[11,12] Mistreatment can impede the positive effects of coming out, with concealment being necessary for safety.[13] However, concealment is associated with reduced social support and increased rates of depression.[13]

Although gender nonconformity poses risk for gender minority stress, this identity is also associated with a number of protective factors that enhance the ability to cope with minority stress and increase resiliency and life meaning. These resilience factors are explored further elsewhere in this article.

## PREVALENCE OF MENTAL DISORDERS IN GENDER DIVERSE CLIENTS

Several studies suggest that TGD individuals experience increased rates of anxiety disorders, bipolar disorder, and depressive disorders, with the latter ranging from 2 to 3 times more prevalent than in the general population.[12,14] Transgender youth in particular have been found to have 2 to 3 times the risk of depressive disorders, anxiety disorders, self-injurious behaviors, suicidal ideation, and suicide attempts.[15] TGD youth are also at least 2 times as likely to be engaged in mental health treatment.

In addition, transgender individuals tend to have an earlier onset of mental disorders.[4,16] This increased prevalence of mental disorders among transgender individuals may contribute to maladaptive strategies to cope with distress, including drug and alcohol abuse, sexual risk taking, and self-injurious behaviors.[6,17–19]

In some cases, the mental health problem may have nothing to do with a person's gender variance, whereas for others, the link may be related to gender dysphoria or transphobia.[7,8] Eating disorders frequently result from efforts to alter one's bodily appearance to conform to social expectations of gender.[20,21] Alternately, the reverse can also be true, such as when gender dysphoria results from psychotic symptomatology.[22] Given that gender dysphoria may enhance mental health problems, alleviation of gender dysphoria may also reduce those mental health concerns through gender affirmation and treatment.[21,23]

Hormone therapy in particular is believed to have a beneficial impact on mental health in enhancing mood, quality of life, and mental wellness.[24] However, some trans women may experience more emotional intensity on estrogen, and trans men may initially feel more emotionally reactive on testosterone.[24] Some research has found that testosterone could have an activating effect on bipolar disorder, requiring close monitoring and adjustment of psychiatric medication.[24] In general, research indicates that hormone therapy tends to boost mood and enhances mental wellness.[25] Mental health providers can provide support to TGD individuals who experience initial adverse changes in mood on hormone therapy. This support might include normalizing changes in mood and providing additional coping strategies such as emotional regulation. The mental health provider should also work in tandem with the prescriber to monitor any negative effects on mood that may require modification, such as a lower and more frequent dosage.[24]

### Depressive Disorders

Depressive symptoms are particularly common among transgender individuals, with rates of depression ranging from 48% to 62% compared with 16.6% in the general population.[5,12,26] One study found depressive symptoms in 51% of trans women and 48% trans men.[26] Although some research finds a relatively equal rate of depression among trans women and trans men,[26] other findings suggest that depression rates may be particularly high for transgender women, who are almost twice as likely as transgender men to meet the criteria for major depressive disorder.[12] In a 3-year prospective study of trans women in New York, major depressive disorder was associated with psychological and physical gender abuse, especially for new or chronic experiences of abuse.[12] This resembles findings in the cisgender populations, where women tend to have higher rates of depression than men, potentially owing to factors such as gender-related abuse and discrimination, as well as gender differences in the experience of and reactions to stress.[27]

Persistent physical abuse and psychological abuse have a clear impact on depression rates among transgender individuals. Psychological abuse is known to contribute to depression in particular, which may be more challenging to psychologically defuse.[12] In a study by Nuttbrock and colleagues,[12] trans women had a 6- to 12-month incidence of depression that was 5 times greater than the general population. In turn, protective socioeconomic factors like employment, income, and education were associated with lower levels depression.

Nuttbrock and colleagues[12] examined the impact of gender-related abuse on depression among trans women across the lifespan. The effects of psychological and physical abuse for major depression was particularly strong during adolescence, and diminished in later phases of life with the use of effective coping strategies for dealing with abuse.

Depression among trans women and their cisgender partners has also been examined.[28] In one study, financial hardship, discrimination, and relationship stigma was associated with an increased likelihood of depressive distress.[28] Approximately 43% of the trans women and 48% of the partners reported clinically significant depression symptoms in the past week. Trans discrimination was correlated with a higher likelihood of depression and lower relationship quality. It seems that stigma takes a toll not only on the trans individual, but on their partners as well, with the financial strain of medical costs or transphobia-related unemployment adding to depression risk.

Related to depression rates is the problem of suicidality. However, although suicidality has been typically treated as a symptom of depression, some suggest that it can take other forms:

1. A separate condition that co-occurs with depression,
2. A condition that arises after a depression has been treated, or
3. A condition that occurs without another underlying mental disorder.[29,30]

The percentage of people with a history of suicidality is very high among TGD individuals.[5,12] In a study of 300 trans participants, 65% reported suicidal ideation—or thoughts of suicide—over the course of their lifetime.[31] Another study of trans women participants found elevated rates of suicidality beyond suicidal ideation (53% transgender; 13% general population), including suicide plans (35%; 3.9%) and suicide attempts (27.9%; 4.6%).[12]

Trans youth may be particularly vulnerable to suicidality. In a study of trans individuals, an attempt was reported in 32% of the total sample, with nearly one-half of the youth in the study reporting a past attempt.[5] In addition to younger age, risk factors for suicide attempts included a history of depression and forced sex, as well as gender-based abuse and victimization.[5] Attempts were particularly greater in the presence of drug and alcohol problems,[32] which may decrease inhibition and increase risk. Gender-based violence also seems to be a key factor in the development of suicidality among transgender individuals.[33] Suicide prevention efforts are underway to address this problem, including transgender suicide hotlines like the Trans Lifeline and the Trevor Project, with the latter directed at lesbian, gay, bisexual, transgender, and queer youth.

### Anxiety Disorders

Estimates of anxiety symptoms among transgender individuals range from 26% to 48% compared with about 29% in the general population.[6,26,34] Anxiety may be a reaction to discrimination and a hypervigilance toward anticipated stigma.[8,13] Anxiety may also result from general life stress, as well challenges with the transition process, peer stigma, sense of loss of social supports, and financial obstacles.[11,12] Devor[35] normalized some anxiety during the early stages of the transition process. This anxiety dissipates with self-acceptance and identity pride, followed by greater well-being in later stages of this process.[11,35] Literature on the prevalence of specific anxiety disorders seems to be limited in at this time. One survey of transgender veterans found 19% indicated that they presented to therapy for a primary problem of anxiety, worry, or panic attacks.[36] More research is needed regarding the occurrence of specific anxiety disorders among TGD individuals.

### Posttraumatic Stress Disorder

Trauma poses risk for not only anxiety and depression but also the development of posttraumatic stress disorder (PTSD).[37] Reisner and colleagues[38] analyzed PTSD rates in a community sample and found them to be much higher than in the general population, even after adjusting for intimate partner violence and childhood abuse. Moreover, this sample experienced worse severity and more emotional numbing, avoidance, and arousal symptoms. Survey participants reported experiencing high levels of discrimination and this discrimination was strongly associated with PTSD.

Higher rates of PTSD may result from increased risk of childhood physical and sexual abuse and intimate partner violence among transgender individuals.[39,40] These statistics may be worsened when one has multiple minority statuses related to racial-ethnic background, income, and sexual orientation.[38] Appearance-related factors may add risk of violence and PTSD, such as high visual gender nonconformity.[38] In addition, Reisner and colleagues[38] found that trans women had higher PTSD rates than trans men, paralleling an increase in PTSD risks among cisgender women. Other predictors of PTSD included childhood abuse, intimate partner violence, depression, and polydrug use. Hence, in a cyclical relationship, the presence of PTSD might increase the likelihood of drug use, which can add further risk of victimization.[41]

### Substance Use Disorders

High rates of substance use disorders among some transgender individuals may reflect an attempt to cope with trauma related to discrimination, as well as other mental health challenges.[9] Estimates of substance use problems range from 10% to 69%,[41,42] and are generally assessed to be higher than in the general population.

Substance use may be related to other risk factors such as unemployment, legal issues, living with a person with a substance abuse problem, and family conflict.[43] Substance use was also associated with physical health problems, and mental health diagnoses.[43] In a study of 155 transgender participants, 26% reported prescription drug abuse, which was associated with clinically significant emotional distress, lower self-esteem, gender identity-related discrimination, anxiety, depression, and somatic symptoms.[44] Thus, the authors believed participants might be self-medicating distress resulting from discrimination.

In another study of trans female youth, drug use was identified as a means of coping with psychological distress.[41] This sample also had high rates of parental drug and alcohol problems, which increased the likelihood of polydrug use and drug use with sex. Similar to other findings,[15] substance use led to additional problems, including high-risk sexual behavior and HIV infection. Consequently, substance use may be involved in a cluster of cooccurring factors, including, depression, discrimination, and high-risk sexual behavior.[42]

## PSYCHOTIC DISORDERS AND SERIOUS MENTAL ILLNESSES

There is a general lack of research on psychotic disorders and serious mental illnesses among transgender individuals. Serious mental illnesses are major mental health disorders that create impairment in at least 2 areas of functioning:

- Occupational/academic/social functioning and self-care, or
- Activities of daily living.

These conditions include schizophrenia spectrum disorders, severe depressive disorders, bipolar disorder, and complex PTSD. One study assessed the incidence of bipolar disorder and schizophrenia to be similar to the general population.[45] A common problem in the treatment of people with psychosis and gender nonconformity is to attribute the gender variance to mental illness and expect "remission" of gender variance with treatment.[22,46] In these cases, transgender identity is often mislabeled as a delusional belief, and providers fear reinforcing a delusion by affirming the person's gender.[22] Other misattributions about gender variance have occurred in the past, including attributing gender identity confusion to schizophrenia,[47] or erroneously labeling transgender identity as essentially "repressed homosexuality."[48]

Mizock and Fleming[??] presented a series of cases that identified variations in the presentation of psychotic disorders and gender nonconformity, including the occurrence of gender variance solely during a psychotic episode, or transgender individuals whose mental illness was distinct from their transgender identity. The authors addressed problems faced by this group, including the tendency of providers to conflate sexual identity and gender identity while overlooking gender variance. Providers charged with discharge plans from inpatient units are often unaware of the potential transphobia-related danger that these clients may face upon transfer to a treatment facility. Some individuals with serious mental illness may also hope that their gender variance will disappear with treatment of their serious mental illness, allowing a return to life without the risk of double stigma and maltreatment. Sensitivity and awareness among clinicians is vital to reducing discriminatory treatment of gender diverse people with serious mental illness to facilitate their recovery.

### Autism Spectrum Disorders

New research is suggesting that gender variance may be higher among individuals with autism spectrum disorders. In a sample of 204 children and adolescents referred for gender dysphoria, the prevalence of autism was 7.8%, up to 37 times more common than in the general population.[49] Another study found a prevalence of 5.5% of gender dysphoria among a sample of individuals with autism, significantly higher than the 0.5% to 2.0% in the general population.[50] Furthermore, estimates of prevalence are complicated by the fact that the symptoms of autism may interfere with a person's ability to articulate their gender identity in some cases.[21,51]

Differences in these rates may occur depending on the birth sex of the individual. Pasterski and colleagues[50] found 7.1% of trans men and 4.8% of trans women had autism, with an average rate of 5.5% for the combined group. Although the research suggests that more people who were assigned males at birth present with autism in childhood, they did not find a significant difference between the gender groups in their study. However, Jones and colleagues[51] found an increase in autism symptom scores in adults with gender dysphoria compared with a comparison group. They also found that trans men presented more autistic traits than did trans women in their sample.

Some case study research suggests that gender variance may be higher among individuals with mild autism spectrum disorder (formerly Asperger's syndrome) as well.[52] Ultimately, the research is still relatively scant in this area, and there is a need for further study and cultural competence in working with gender diversity among neurodiverse populations.

### Eating Disorders

Several studies have addressed the presentation of eating disorders and body image problems among some transgender individuals.[53,54] These problems tend to reflect gender pressures related to sexism in the cisgender population, and therefore seem to be influenced by gender expression among transgender individuals as well.[20,21,55] For example, cases of anorexia and bulimia have been reported among transgender women as attempts to achieve a feminine body shape and with the added pressure to achieve traditional feminine beauty ideals of thinness.[53] Other case studies have discussed eating problems among trans men that occurred to achieve a masculine or boyish physique, or to reduce chest size and curves.[54]

Modulation of menstruation has also been identified as a factor in eating disorders in this group. Trans men might develop anorexia to stop menstruation, and in turn, trans women might attribute anorexia-related emaciation as a justification for the lack of menstruation.[55] In addition, some research suggests that gender affirmation procedures may alleviate gender dysphoria-based eating problems.[20] The onset of an eating disorder can be triggered by major life changes and stressors.[54] Some individuals undergoing a gender affirmation process may experience stress related to a major life change or increased risk of transphobia. Therefore, mental health providers should assess for eating disordered behavior during the gender affirmation process. Additional research is needed in this area to fully assess prevalence and culturally responsive treatment strategies.

## RESILIENCE

TGD individuals draw from a number of important resilience factors to overcome the effects of transphobia.[13] For one, religious or spiritual beliefs have been associated with resilience and reduced levels of depression, so long as these practices enable positive coping behaviors and social support. Some trans individuals experience stigma in their religious communities. Religious communities that offer social support can enhance resilience.

Self-esteem has also been found to predict depression scores among transgender participants.[13] Transgender identity pride and acceptance of gender identity may increase well-being later on and act as a further buffer against minority stress, protecting against transphobia-related depression.[56] Social support and family support seem to be important protective mental health factors in particular.[8,57] Research has found that peer support is associated with lower levels of depression, particularly for trans youth.[13] Social support might take place through social media, support groups, and involvement in activist communities.

Relatedly, positive mental health effects are associated with hormone therapy. Research has found positive effects of hormone treatment on mood, cognitive function, well-being, emotional stability, and health-related quality of life.[25] Trans men who receive testosterone have reported lower levels of depression, anxiety, irritability, and stress.[25] Meier and colleagues[25] suggested that any initial emotional reactivity related to hormone therapy was generally offset by long-term gains. Based on these findings, the authors discouraged withholding hormone therapy or gender affirmation surgeries based on suicide risk or depression history.

Coping strategies are key protective factors in reducing the impact of psychological distress from external and internalized stigma.[8] Evidence suggests that some types of coping strategies are more effective than others, such as active or problem-focused coping skills, which have been found to reduce mental health problems like depression.[58] Avoidant coping has been found to decrease over the course of transition, with more active coping used during and after transition, potentially leading to lower levels of distress during these times.[58]

## TREATMENT RECOMMENDATIONS

The prevalence of depression, anxiety, suicide, anxiety, PTSD, substance abuse, and eating disorders suggest the need to screen for these conditions among transgender individuals. The complexity of autism and psychosis in the presence of gender variance requires the need for astute differential diagnosis. Members of the treatment team should be mindful of any possible drug interactions with the use of hormone therapy and psychotropic medications in the treatment of mental disorders. Assessment should be conducted to evaluate the impact of mental health problems on maladaptive behaviors such as substance use, which may reflect a means to cope with psychological distress. Exploration of the effects of transphobia and gender minority stress on transgender individuals is also warranted. Taking an intersectionality perspective on the multiple, overlapping identities that may contribute to added oppression is needed, such as in the case of trans people who experience oppression related to race/ethnicity, disability, poverty, and other factors. The focus on psycho-pathology can be balanced with examination of sources of support, resilience, and coping strategies.

Transgender individuals can be supported to enhance coping strategies and social supports in psychotherapy. The impact of the gender affirmation process and hormone therapy on one's mental health should also be addressed, recognizing that these processes could facilitate mental wellness. Support groups can be a particularly valuable avenue for maximizing social support and enhancing resilience.

Psychotherapy recommendations have also been suggested in a study investigating problems faced by transgender individuals in psychotherapy. Therapists might make errors in overemphasizing, underemphasizing, or stigmatizing gender diverse identities in psychotherapy sessions.[59] Psychotherapists might place the burden of education on the client, overassert power, or perform care in a perfunctory manner. Moreover, it is unlikely that one particular psychotherapy approach is best suited for working with transgender individuals. As with any therapeutic orientation, each approach may have its unique benefits depending on the particular problem at hand and preference of the individual client. Regardless of therapeutic orientation, it is important that the mental health provider follows culturally responsive recommendations for care, such as in the aforementioned study on therapist missteps and the American Psychological Association guidelines.[21] Ultimately, sensitivity to mental health problems faced by gender diverse individuals is essential to overcoming mental health challenges and promoting resilience.

## SUMMARY

The presentation of mental disorders among TGD individuals is largely impacted by transphobia and gender-related discrimination and abuse. Anxiety, distress, and other mental health challenges might also be affected by initial gender dysphoria, which is often resolved with gender affirmation and culturally competent care and treatment. Political and social change is needed to help reduce transphobia and the associated gender minority stress that contributes to mental health concerns. Providers can help to develop policy and programs that promote resilience and well-being in the trans community through the delivery of gender-responsive care.

## REFERENCES

1. Perone AK. The social construction of mental illness for lesbian, gay, bisexual, and transgender persons in the United States. Qual Soc Work 2014;13(6): 766–71.
2. Lev AI. Gender dysphoria: two steps forward, one step back. Clin Soc Work J 2013;41(3):288–96.
3. Perlick DA, Nelson AH, Mattias K, et al. In our own voice–family companion: Reducing self-stigma of family members of persons with serious mental illness. Psychiatr Serv 2011;62(12):1456–62.
4. Kidd SA, Veltman A, Gately C, et al. Lesbian, gay, and transgender persons with severe mental illness: negotiating wellness in the context of multiple sources of stigma. Am J Psychiatr Rehabil 2011;14:13–39.
5. Clements-Nolle K, Marx R, Katz M. Attempted suicide among transgender persons. J Homosex 2006;51(3):53–69.

6. Mustanski BS, Garofalo R, Emerson EM. Mental health disorders, psychological distress, and suicidality in a diverse sample of lesbian, gay, bisexual, and transgender youths. Am J Public Health 2010;100:2426–32.

7. Hendricks ML, Testa RJ. A conceptual framework for clinical work with transgender and gender nonconforming clients: an adaptation of the minority stress model. Prof Psychol Res Pract 2012;43:460–7.

8. Meyer IH. Prejudice, social stress, and mental health in lesbian, gay, and bisexual populations: conceptual issues and research evidence. Psychol Bull 2003; 129(5):674–97.

9. Grant JM, Mottet LA, Tanis J, et al. Injustice at every turn: a report of the national transgender discrimination survey. Washington, DC: National Center for Transgender Equality and National Gay and Lesbian Task Force; 2011.

10. Lombardi EL, Wilchins RA, Priesing D, et al. Gender violence: transgender experiences with violence and discrimination. J Homosex 2001;42:89–101.

11. Budge SL, Adelson JL, Howard KAS. Anxiety and depression in transgender individuals: the roles of transition status, loss, social support, and coping. J Consult Clin Psychol 2013;81(3):545–57.

12. Nuttbrock L, Bockting W, Rosenblum A, et al. Gender abuse and major depression among transgender women: a prospective study of vulnerability and resilience. American Journal of Public Health 2014;104(11):2191–8.

13. Merryman M, Mizock L. LGBTQ depression. In: Goldberg A, editor. Thousand Oaks (CA): Sage Encyclopedia of LGBTQ Studies; 2016. p. 297–301.

14. McDuffie E, Brown G. 70 US veterans with gender identity disturbances: a descriptive study. Int J Transgend 2010;12(1):21–30.

15. Reisner SL, Vetters R, Leclerc M, et al. Discriminatory experiences associated with posttraumatic stress disorder symptoms among transgender adults. J Adolesc Health 2015;56(3):274–9.

16. Hellman RE, Sudderth L, Avery AM. Major mental illness in a sexual minority psychiatric sample. J Gay Lesbian Med Assoc 2002;6:97–106.

17. Garofalo R, Deleon J, Osmer E, et al. Overlooked, misunderstood, and at risk: exploring the lives and HIV risk of ethnic minority male-to-female transgender youth. J Adolesc Health 2006;38:230–6.

18. Liu RT, Mustanski B. Suicidal ideation and self-harm in lesbian, gay, bisexual, and transgender youth. Am J Prev Med 2012;42:221–8.

19. Reisner SL, Perkovich B, Mimiaga M. A mixed methods study of the sexual health needs of New England trans men who have sex with nontransgender men. AIDS Patient Care STDs 2010;24:501–13.

20. Ålgars M, Alanko K, Santilla P, et al. Disordered eating and Gender Identity Disorder: a qualitative study. Eat Disord 2012;20:300–11.

21. American Psychological Association. Guidelines for psychological practice with transgender and gender nonconforming people. Washington, DC: Author; 2015.

22. Mizock L, Fleming M. Transgender and gender variant populations with mental illness: implications for clinical care. Prof Psychol 2011;42(2):208–13.

23. Keo-Meier CL, Herman LI, Reisner SL, et al. Testosterone treatment and MMPI-2 improvement in transgender men: a prospective controlled study. J Consult Clin Psychol 2015;83(1):143–56.

24. Coleman E, Bockting W, Botzer M, et al. Standards of care for the health of transsexual, transgender, and gender nonconforming people, 7th version. Int J Transgend 2012;13:165–232.

25. Meier SC, Fitzgerald KM, Pardo ST, et al. The effects of hormonal gender affirmation treatment on mental health in female-to-male transsexuals. J Gay Lesbian Ment Health 2011;15(3):281–99.

26. Kessler RC, Berglund P, Demler O, et al. Lifetime prevalence and age of onset distributions of DSM-IV disorders in the national comorbidity survey replication. Arch Gen Psychiatry 2005;62:593–602.

27. Nolen-Hoeksema S. Gender differences in depression. Curr Dir Psychol Sci 2014; 10(5):173–6.

28. Gamarel KE, Reisner SL, Laurenceau J, et al. Gender minority stress, mental health, and relationship quality: an investigation of transgender women and their cisgender male partners. J Fam Psychol 2014;28(4):437–47.

29. Colt GH. November of the soul: the enigma of suicide. New York: Simon and Schuster; 2006.

30. Solomon A. The noonday demon: an atlas of depression. New York: Simon and Schuster; 2011.

31. Xavier J, Honnold JA, Bradford J. The health, health-related needs, and life-course experiences of transgender Virginians. Richmond (VA): Virginia Department of Health; 2007.

32. Mathy RM. Transgender identity and suicidality in a nonclinical sample: sexual orientation, psychiatric history, and compulsive behaviors. J Psychol Human Sex 2012;14(4):47–65.

33. Goldblum P, Testa RJ, Pflum S, et al. The relationship between gender-based victimization and suicide attempts in transgender people. Prof Psychol Res Pract 2012;43(5):468–75.

34. Hepp U, Kraemer B, Schnyder U, et al. Psychiatric comorbidity in gender identity disorder. J Psychosom Res 2005;58:259–61.

35. Devor AH. Witnessing and mirroring: a fourteen stage model of transsexual identity formation. J Gay Lesb Psychother 2004;8:41–67.

36. Shipherd JC, Green K, Abramovitz S. Transgender clients: identifying and minimizing barriers to mental health treatment. J Gay Lesbian Ment Health 2010; 14:94–108.

37. Mizock L, Lewis TK. Trauma in transgender populations: risk, resilience, and clinical care. J Emot Abuse 2008;8(3):335–54.

38. Reisner SL, White JM, Gamarel KE, et al. Discriminatory experiences associated with posttraumatic stress disorder symptoms among transgender adults. J Couns Psychol 2016;63(5):509–19.

39. Brewin CR, Andrews B, Valentine JD. Meta-analysis of risk factors for posttraumatic stress disorder in trauma-exposed adults. J Consult Clin Psychol 2000; 68:748–66.

40. Golding JM. Intimate partner violence as a risk factor for mental disorders: a meta-analysis. J Fam Violence 1999;14:99–132.

41. Rowe C, Santos G, McFarland W, et al. Prevalence and correlates of substance use among trans*female youth ages 16-24 years in the San Francisco Bay Area. Drug Alcohol Depend 2015;147:160–6.

42. Keuroghlian AS, Reisner SL, White JM, et al. Substance use and treatment of substance use disorders in a community sample of transgender adults. Drug Alcohol Depend 2015;152:139–46.

43. Flentje A, Heck NC, Sorensen JL. Characteristics of transgender individuals entering substance abuse treatment. Addict Behav 2014;39:969–75.

44. Benotsch EG, Zimmerman R, Cathers L, et al. Non-medical use of prescription drugs, polysubstance use, and mental health in transgender adults. Drug Alcohol Depend 2013;132:391–4.
45. Cole CM, O'Boyle M, Emory LE, et al. Comorbidity of gender dysphoria and other major psychiatric diagnoses. Arch Sex Behav 1997;26(1):13–26.
46. Baltieri DA, De Andrade AG. Schizophrenia Modifying the expression of gender identity disorder. J Sex Med 2009;6:1185–8.
47. Latorre RA, Endman M, Gossmann I. Androgyny and need achievement in male and female psychiatric inpatients. J Clin Psychol 1976;32:232–5.
48. Socarides C. The desire for sexual transformation: a psychiatric evaluation of transsexualism. Am J Psychiatry 1969;125:1419–25.
49. deVries ALC, Noens ILJ, Cohen-Kettenis PT, et al. Autism spectrum disorders in gender dysphoric children and adolescents. J Autism Dev Disord 2010;40:930–6.
50. Pasterski V, Gilligan L, Curtis R. Traits of autism spectrum disorders in adults with gender dysphoria. Arch Sex Behav 2014;43:387–93.
51. Jones RM, Wheelwright S, Farrell K, et al. Brief report: female-to-male transsexual people and autistic traits. J Autism Dev Disord 2012;42:301–6.
52. Parkinson J. Gender dysphoria in Asperger's syndrome: a caution. Australas Psychiatry 2014;22(1):84–5.
53. Vocks S, Stahn C, Loenser L, et al. Eating and body image disturbances in male-to-female and female-to-male transsexuals. Arch Sex Behav 2009;38:364–77.
54. Strandjord SE, Ng H, Rome ES. Effects of treating gender dysphoria and anorexia nervosa in a transgender adolescent: lessons learned. Int J Eat Disord 2015; 48(7):942–5.
55. Murray SB, Boon E, Touyz SW. Diverging eating psychopathology in transgendered eating disorder patients: a report of two cases. Eat Disord 2013; 21(1):70–4.
56. Singh A, Hays D, Watson L. Strength in the face of adversity: resilience strategies of transgender individuals. J Couns Dev 2011;89:20–7.
57. Ryan C, Huebner D, Diaz RM, et al. Family rejection as a predictor of negative health outcomes in White and Latino lesbian, gay and bisexual young adults. Pediatrics 2009;123(1):346–52.
58. Budge SL, Katz-Wise SL, Tebbe E, et al. Transgender emotional and coping processes: use of facilitative and avoidant coping throughout the gender transition. Couns Psychol 2013;41:601–47.
59. Mizock L, Lundquist C. Missteps in psychotherapy with transgender clients: promoting gender sensitivity in counseling and psychological practice. Psychology of Sexual Orientation and Gender Diversity 2016;3(2):148–55.

# Treatment of Trauma and Nonsuicidal Self-Injury in Transgender Adults

lore m. dickey, PhD[a],*, Anneliese A. Singh, PhD[b],
Daniel Walinsky, PhD[c]

## KEYWORDS

- Transgender - Gender diverse - Trauma - Nonsuicidal self-injury - Rapport

## KEY POINTS

- Mental health providers must explore the ways trauma and nonsuicidal self-injury (NSI) have impacted the lives of transgender people.
- Mental health providers must assess for and treat trauma and NSI.
- Neither trauma nor NSI need be a contraindication to a social or medical transition.
- Mental health providers must build a strong working alliance or rapport with their clients.
- Mental health providers are encouraged to ensure that client's mental health concerns are reasonably well-controlled.

Transgender and gender nonconforming (TGNC) adults experience high rates of trauma and nonsuicidal self-injury (NSI). In a survey of more than 6000 participants, 41% of transgender respondents indicated that they had attempted suicide at least once.[1] The rates of suicide attempts for this participant group increased when there were experiences of employment discrimination and job loss (55%), school bullying (51%), and physical and sexual assault (61% and 64%, respectively). Many researchers have suggested that the high rates of transgender suicide attempts are linked to experiences of minority stress.[2–4] Minority stress has been defined as chronic stress related to discrimination that leads to concealment of transgender identity, internalization of trans-negative beliefs and attitudes, and anticipation of antitransgender discrimination.[5,6]

Disclosure Statement: None of the authors have a conflict of interest nor are we receiving any funding for this work.

a Department of Educational Psychology, Northern Arizona University, 801 South Knoles Drive, Building 27A, Room 110, PO Box 5774, Flagstaff, AZ 86011-5774, USA; b Department of Counseling & Human Development Services, The University of Georgia, 402 Aderhold Hall, Athens, GA 30602-7142, USA; c Psychology Department, Salem State University, 352 Lafayette Street, Salem, MA 0970, USA
* Corresponding author.
E-mail address: lore.dickey@nau.edu

Psychiatr Clin N Am 40 (2017) 41–50
http://dx.doi.org/10.1016/j.psc.2016.10.007
0193-953X/17/© 2016 Elsevier Inc. All rights reserved.

| Abbreviations | |
|---|---|
| NSI | Nonsuicidal self-injury |
| PTSD | Posttraumatic stress disorder |
| TGNC | Transgender and gender nonconforming |

This minority stress can also lead to high rates of NSI. Some people who use NSI as a means of coping do so in a manner to address actual or perceived stressors. dickey and Garza[7] found that gender diverse people use NSI in ways that are different than the general population. Specifically, resilience is seen to be a means of coping; that gender diverse people use ways of coping to rise above the challenges they face on a daily basis. In addition to increased NSI, there are health disparities related to rates of trauma for transgender adults. In 2013, transgender women comprised 72% of hate crime murders and were nearly twice as likely to experience sexual violence than cisgender women. A compounding issue is that transgender people may not seek assistance from institutions to cope with these traumatic events, and when they do seek these services they are likely to experience harm from the very people who are supposed to protect them. For instance, this same survey found that transgender people were 7 times more likely to experience police violence in their interactions with police. In this article, the different forms of trauma that transgender people experience are described and how transgender people can have traumatic experiences when accessing necessary transgender-related health care. Special attention is given to NSI that transgender adults experience. A discussion of how to work with transgender people within a trauma context is also provided.

## TRANSGENDER ADULTS AND EXPERIENCES OF TRAUMA

Trauma is a term encompassing a variety of experiences that can cause psychological, physical, and sexual harm. Intimate partner violence, sexual assault, and child sexual abuse are some examples of trauma that transgender people may experience. The Centers for Disease Control and Prevention[8] define traumatic events as those that "are marked by a sense of horror, helplessness, serious injury, or the threat of serious injury or death" (p. 1). In the *Diagnostic and Statistical Manual of Mental Disorders* posttraumatic stress disorder (PTSD) is defined as a person having experienced or witnessed a traumatic even and, having done so, the individual is experiencing symptoms that are causing distress.[9] Mental health practitioners working with transgender people should be especially cognizant of how trauma can influence overall health and well-being owing to the high rates of trauma that transgender adults have.[10] Mental health practitioners should be trained in lifespan approaches, because the types of trauma transgender adults may experience can influence developmental milestones and the overall life course. In addition, mental health practitioners must seek to understand the history of trauma that transgender people have experienced within health care institutions, including counseling and psychology, to most effectively serve transgender clients. Each of these areas is discussed in relation to transgender people and trauma.

### Assessing Trauma

Trauma is culturally bound and influenced by society, so a socioecological approach can be helpful when assessing transgender clients.[11] Socioecological models bring attention to the various levels that might influence an individual's life. The Centers for Disease Control and Prevention[12] use a 4-level socioecological model to focus intervention and prevention work: individual, relationship, community, and societal levels. It can also be helpful to expand and refine the potential levels of the socioeco-logical model, such as defining how the intrapersonal, interpersonal, institutional, community, public policy, and international levels[13] influence the trauma that trans-gender people experience. For instance, transgender people may experience intra-personal trauma (eg, negative self-talk, maladaptive coping) or they may experience interpersonal trauma within relationships (eg, intimate partner violence). Transgender people can experience microaggressions related to their gender, which are everyday lived experiences of transnegativity they experience (eg, being asked if they have had "the" surgery or being misgendered by people using the wrong pronouns or names to refer to them).[14]

Transgender people may also experience trauma within societal institutions, such educational settings where they may not be able to use the bathrooms of their choice or may experience school bullying and harassment. At the community level, trans-gender adults are subject to community norms that are often trans-negative and dis-affirming of transgender people. These community norms are upheld by individual members of society and can include stereotypes and biases toward transgender peo-ple. At the public policy level, there are laws and policies (eg, local, state, federal) that can be sites of trauma for transgender people, such as the bathroom law passed by North Carolina in 2015 that bans transgender people from using the bathroom that is consistent with their affirmed gender. Finally, international levels of trauma for trans-gender people can include the stories of discrimination and violence that are experi-enced by transgender people around the world, such as the violence that transgender people in Brazil experience.[15]

In addition to considering the pervasiveness of these multiple levels of trauma, mental health practitioners should be well-versed in diagnosis with trauma. For instance, PTSD may be a common diagnosis that transgender people have owing to the extensive context of trauma.[10] At the same time, mental health practitioners should be aware of the common sources of PTSD that transgender people may report to not only accurately diagnose PTSD (and complex PTSD as well), but also to be able to assess the sources of trauma. Although some traumatic experiences may lead to a diagnosis of PTSD, not all do. Unless a person is experiencing distress as a result of their traumatic experience(s), no diagnosis is warranted.[9] Further, traumatic experi-ences may lead to other mental health concerns (eg, depression, anxiety). In a study of more than 400 transgender adults examining transgender people and PTSD symp-toms found that participants identified 5 sources of discrimination, including their gender identity and gender expression, appearance as masculine or feminine, sexual orientation, sex assigned at birth, and age.[10] Study authors recommended that mental health practitioners must endeavor to conduct a thorough trauma assessment at intake and throughout counseling owing to the high rates of trauma in transgender communities.

## Transgender Trauma and Lifespan Considerations

Much of the trauma experiences, symptoms, and levels in which trauma is experi-enced for transgender people influences the developmental milestones and life course of this group because of the pervasiveness of trauma. For some transgender adults, they may be able to trace the influence of trans-negative environments within their early childhood experiences. They may report that they were admonished or experi-enced even worse consequences for gender expansive behaviors[17] from families, school personnel, and/or communities (eg, places of worship). Adolescence can also be a time in the lifespan of considerable vulnerability. A considerable body of research has documented the influence of school bullying and violence on the lives of gender diverse young people.[18–20] Adolescents are exploring their place in the world, and if they are not allowed to explore their gender with family support, they may report negative effects on their development (eg, dating violence, internalized shame).

In early and middle adulthood, trauma can additionally occur within work settings. Transgender people may be exploring their gender identity and expression for the first time and experience workplace violence or rejection within their families when they disclose their gender identities. For other transgender people in early and middle adulthood, they may have begun their own families or had children before they identified as transgender and may experience the loss of relationships, marriages, and custody when they disclose their transgender identity. In older adulthood, transgender people who have lived their lives in the gender they know themselves to be may feel forced to conceal their transgender identity or experience a lack of support and respect for their gender identity when they access assisted living, hospice care, or other older adult settings.

### Trauma Within Health Care Settings

Each of the experiences across the lifespan discussed comes with not only the impact of trauma, but also experiences of trauma that are chronic, persistent, and focused on a singular part of their identity, which can make transgender adults feel weary and suspicious of working with mental health practitioners. Therefore, it is critical that mental health practitioners be well-informed of transgender-affirmative care when they are providing trauma-informed approaches with transgender clients. Transgender-affirming mental health care is defined as "culturally-relevant for TGNC clients and their multiple social identities, addresses the influence of social inequities on the lives of TGNC clients, enhances TGNC client resilience and coping, advocates to reduce systemic barriers to TGNC mental and physical health, and leverages TGNC client strengths."[21]

Attending to these components of transgender-affirming care requires an awareness of the common distrust that transgender adults can bring into the counseling session with them. For decades, the transgender community has been told when, how, and where they can access transgender-related health care. The gatekeeping role of mental health practitioners has, therefore, been reinforced over time, where transgender people may not feel in control of their health care treatment. A shift in this gatekeeping role has been encouraged, moving to centralize mental health practitioner advocacy as crucial to providing effective treatment with transgender clients.[22] Mental health practitioners can acknowledge, validate, and explore this natural distrust that is the result of what transgender communities have experienced with health care providers and what they may have heard from community members. Addressing this potential distrust directly, communicating an explicit approach to care that is trans affirming, and engaging in advocacy for TGNC people that can strengthen rapport building and help to build a collaborative relationship between provider and client. This collaborative relationship is crucial because the counseling relationship has the potential to be one of the few places that transgender clients experience the space to heal and be free from traumatic events.

## TRANSGENDER ADULTS AND NONSUICIDAL SELF-INJURY

NSI can be a complicated mental health concern that may lead to the need for extensive clinical treatment. Historically, NSI has been associated with borderline personality disorder.[9] In the *Diagnostic and Statistical Manual of Mental Disorders* (5th ed)[9] NSI is listed as a condition for further study. NSI includes a variety of behaviors (eg, cutting, interfering with wound healing, burning) in which a person engages without a lethal intent.[23] Rates of NSI in the general public are from 1% to 23%.[24] dickey and colleagues[25] found that 42% of transgender people in their study had a history of NSI. The study also found that gender nonbinary and trans masculine participants were at greater risk for NSI than trans feminine participants. One of the manners in which people engage in NSI (sticking themselves with needles) was elevated as compared with the general population. This finding was especially interesting considering that some TGNC people use needles and syringes for administration of hormones. The results of this study elucidate the need to explore NSI in gender diverse people because this may be an important clinical consideration.

### Assessing Nonsuicidal Self-injury in Gender Diverse People

Gender diverse people often face a variety of challenges that have the potential to complicate their mental health. Some people may use NSI as a means of coping with these challenges. dickey and Garza[7] found that the Depression Anxiety Stress Scale[26,27] and the Body Investment Scale[28] were both predictive of NSI. It is important to determine a cutoff score for these scales at which a person's risk for NSI can be more accurately determined. Even though this cutoff information does not exist currently exist, providers are encouraged to use the Depression Anxiety Stress Scale and the Body Investment Scale as elements of their clinical assessment when determining readiness for a social or medical transition. If a client has elevated scores on the Depression Anxiety Stress Scale or low scores on the Body Investment Scale (low scores are indicative of a low investment in one's body) further inquiry about the client's history of NSI would be appropriate.

Clients with a history of NSI may or may not be ready for a social or medical transition. There is no literature that explores the ways that gender diverse people engage in NSI as they commence their transition. The World Professional Association for Transgender Health Standards of Care[29] discuss the importance of ensuring that mental health concerns are "reasonably well-controlled" (p. 104). This does not mean that NSI needs to be absent from a person's life, rather that the client has some coping mechanisms that are strengths based and adaptive.[25] NSI is commonly seen as a maladaptive coping mechanism. For transgender and gender diverse people who experience interpersonal and intrapersonal stressors, it is important to ensure that clients are engaging in mindfulness activities that can help to reduce the impact of these stressors.

### Transgender Nonsuicidal Self-injury and Lifespan Considerations

NSI often first appears in adolescence.[23,30] This is true in the general population as well as for gender diverse people.[25] There are no data that clearly show whether there is a link between a person initiating NSI and coming to terms with their gender diverse identity. The earlier a gender diverse person initiates NSI, the more likely they are to continue engaging in this behavior.[7] Further, dickey[31] found that 50% of gender diverse people with a history NSI stopped this behavior 2 years before starting transition. Nearly 80% of participants reported having stopped NSI within 1 year after beginning transition; this number increases to 92.8% within 5 years of initiating transition and to 97% after 10 years.[31] Further research is needed to understand the differences between those people who stop engaging in NSI and those who do not.

Some providers are reluctant to make a referral for a medical transition for gender diverse people who are deemed to have cooccurring mental health concerns. NSI is one such clinical concern. Given that research show that gender diverse people stop engaging in NSI both before and after transition, NSI should not be assumed to be a contraindication to transition. It is difficult to say whether the timing around the cessation of NSI is related the natural aging process in which people are assumed to stop NSI as they move into adulthood, if NSI and one's gender diverse identity are connected, or if the fact that some providers essentially prevent a social or medical transition until cooccurring mental health concerns have been resolved.

These questions about NSI and gender diverse people warrant further research. There is a need for research that explores the ways that NSI coincides with a person's exploration of their gender and how and if NSI abates when a person initiates a social or medical transition. One should not immediately assume that the presence of NSI is a reason to prevent the commencement of a gender diverse person's transition process. Providers are encouraged to explore the triggers that lead to NSI and the functions that NSI serve for their clients. Further, it is critical that providers work with their clients to ensure that the clients have a variety of strengths-based coping strategies.[25,31]

## DISCUSSION

Clinical work with transgender and gender diverse people can be complicated by the history of gatekeeping for which the mental health field is known.[32] Given that many transgender people are required to access mental health care by medical providers or insurance companies, it is critical that providers be well-informed and have the ability to create a positive working relationship. In this section, we explore the ways in which providers might address rapport in the clinical setting. We also explore the concept of reasonably well-controlled. Given that some providers are reluctant to support a social or medical transition, it is important to understand how these ideas impact the clinical relationship.

### Rapport

Building rapport with clients is a task that is done early in therapy and is foundational to building a therapeutic alliance and, therefore, to providing effective trauma therapy. Several considerations for effectively building rapport with TGNC people, especially in context of providing trauma therapy should be considered.

Before meeting with clients, there are steps that clinicians and mental health professionals can take to support effective rapport building with TGNC clients. First, clinicians should build their knowledge base about issues that impact the local and national transgender communities. They should also learn about local, regional, and national resources for TGNC people, so that they are able to provide appropriate support, resources, and referrals. Additionally, mental health professionals should explore and understand their own gender identity development in the context of salient identities that lead to marginalization or benefit within interlocking systems of cisgenderism (the assumption that all people are cisgender and the ways in which cisgender people are privileged), sexism, racism, heterosexism, ableism, and classism. Inherent in this process of identity exploration is understanding the historical gatekeeping role that mental health providers have traditionally played in the process of accessing gender-affirming medical and surgical interventions. Clinicians should be aware of how this history—and the ongoing role of letter writers who support access to transition-related services—may naturally inhibit trust as clinical work begins. Therefore, clinicians should not immediately judge clients who do not fully disclose symptoms of gender dysphoria or negative coping strategies (eg, NSI, substance abuse) as being resistant or consider their lack of full disclosure as evidence of more severe psychopathology. Rather, they should understand that a client who understands the gatekeeping role of a mental health provider may be trying to present themselves in the most positive way to ensure access to needed medical and surgical services.

Efforts to provide a safe environment are necessary for building positive rapport, regardless of whether a client has experienced a recent and acute trauma (eg, an assault, car accident, witnessing physical violence), or is experiencing the impact of ongoing, repetitive microaggresions, or insidious identity-based trauma.[33] To this end, efforts can be made on both the environmental and interpersonal levels to build safety and trust. For example, environmental interventions such as visual cues that affirm gender, racial, and ethnic diversity (eg, signs and posters), and trans-affirming paperwork (eg, including qualitative response for gender markers, as opposed to check boxes)[34] may help TGNC people to feel support as they come to a clinic or office for the first time. Such visible signs of support may be especially important for TGNC people who have recently experienced a trauma. For any marginalized group, finding representations of their cultural background and experience can be welcoming.

Beyond environmental cues, interpersonal interactions with staff help to build positive rapport. For example, using appropriate pronouns helps to demonstrate care and understanding and may reduce the potential for retraumatization through misgendering. Additionally, deeper work done by cisgender staff can also contribute to building positive rapport. Cisgender mental health professionals who work with TGNC clients should understand their own gender identity, developmentally and contextually,[34] and have a fluent understanding of both binary and fluid constructs of gender. Such an understanding will help staff to speak knowledgably about gender identity with all clients, and particularly with TGNC clients. Furthermore, given the nearly ubiquitous experience of discrimination reported by TGNC people,[1] mental health providers should be able to recognize some of the common manifestations of insidious trauma experiences and posttraumatic stress that may develop after repetitive trans-negative interactions that can occur within family, workplace, and social settings.

### Reasonably Well-Controlled

For professionals who follow the World Professional Association for Transgender Health Standards of Care,[29] access to transition-related services is contingent on medical and mental health concerns of TGNC clients being "reasonably well-controlled." Given the importance of access to transition-related services for some TGNC people, accurately assessing mental health concerns is vital.[34] An accurate assessment requires an understanding of differential diagnosis that accounts for the symptom manifestation of various types of common and insidious identity-related traumas,[33] along with symptoms of concurrent mental health conditions, such as anxiety and depression that are common among trauma survivors. To accurately assess the extent to which a mental health concern is reasonably well-controlled, it is vital to understand such concerns contextually, and to provide appropriate support.

It is important to consider individual as well as contextual and environmental factors in assessing the extent to which a mental health condition is "reasonably well-controlled,"[29] For example, it is essential to understand individual coping strategies, along with presence or absence of negative or positive symptoms. Similarly, given that the vast majority of TGNC people have reported identity-related discrimination[1] experiences of minority stress,[4] insidious trauma should be considered. Given the multiple and pervasive presence of interpersonal and environmental stressors such as a lack of safety in restrooms, difficulty in accessing transition-related services, and disproportionate trans-negative interpersonal violence,[1,33] a reasonably well-controlled mental health condition is highly unlikely to mean an absence of all mental health symptoms. Rather, it is important to balance severity of symptoms, the potential for reduction of symptoms after identity-affirming interventions (eg, social and/or medical transition), differential identity-based experiences (eg, binary or fluid identity, intersections of trans-negativity, racism, classism, heterosexism, sexism), and the coping skills that clients are able to access. Further, mental health providers should understand the ways in which behaviors such as NSI may be used as coping strategies[25] and are not evidence of a poorly controlled mental health condition.

Evidence strongly suggests that accessing gender-affirming medical services, such as hormone therapy, can help to reduce negative mental health symptoms among TGNC people.[35] As mental health providers conceptualize clinical work with TGNC people who have experienced trauma and who are seeking gender-affirming services, they should consider evidence-based approaches that integrate the best available research with clinical judgment to assess the likelihood of symptom reduction after gender-affirming intervention. From this perspective, as mental health provider do trauma work with a TGNC client for whom gender-affirming medical and/or surgical interventions are likely to reduce symptoms of gender dysphoria, it is appropriate to assume that symptoms of gender dysphoria will continue to be present—to some degree—until that person can access appropriate care. During this process, clients can benefit from building positive coping strategies to best manage the impact of negative interpersonal and environmental stressors.

## SUMMARY

Gender diverse people may engage in clinical services as the result of the desire to make a social or medical transition. Mental health providers are often placed in a tenuous position when they are asked to provide a letter of support to a medical provider. This places the mental health provider in the place of significant power, which may be perceived by the client as unnecessarily obstructing a client's process for affirming their gender. Mental health providers are encouraged to explore trauma and NSI in their client's clinical history without assuming that the presence of these clinical concerns prevents a client from initiating a social or medical transition.

## REFERENCES

1. Grant JM, Mottet LA, Tanis J, et al. Injustice at every turn: a report of the national transgender discrimination survey. 2011. Available at: http://endtransdiscrimination.org/PDFs/NTDS_Report.pdf. Accessed July 22, 2016.
2. Blosnich JR, Brown GR, Shipherd JC, et al. Prevalence of gender identity disorder and suicide risk among transgender veterans utilizing Veterans' Health Administration care. Am J Public Health 2013;103(10):e27–32.
3. Mizock L, Mueser KT. Employment, mental health, internalized stigma, and coping with transphobia among transgender individuals. Psychol Sex Orientat Gend Divers 2014;1(2):146–58.
4. Hendricks ML, Testa RJ. A conceptual framework for clinical work with transgender and gender nonconforming clients: an adaptation of the minority stress model. Prof Psychol Res Pr 2012;43:460–7.
5. Meyer IH. Minority stress and mental health in gay men. J Health Soc Behav 1995;36:38–56.
6. Meyer IH. Prejudice, social stress, and mental health in lesbian, gay, and bisexual populations: conceptual issues and research evidence. Psychol Bull 2003;129:674–97.

7. dickey lm, Garza MV. Nonsuicidal self-injury in the transgender community: an international sample. Paper presented at the International Congress of Psychology. Yokohama (Japan), July 27, 2016.
8. Centers for Disease Control and Prevention. Coping with a traumatic event. Available at: http://www.cdc.gov/masstrauma/factsheets/public/coping.pdf. Accessed on July 22, 2016.
9. American Psychiatric Association. Diagnostic and statistical manual of mental disorders. 5th edition. Washington, DC: Author; 2013.
10. Richmond K, Burnes TR, Singh AA, et al. Assessment and treatment of trauma with transgender and gender nonconforming clients: a feminist approach. In: Singh AA, dickey lm, editors. Affirmative counseling and psychological practice with transgender and gender nonconforming clients. Washington, DC: American Psychological Association; 2016. p. 191–212.
11. Institute of Medicine. The health of lesbian, gay, bisexual, and transgender people: building a foundation for better understanding. Washington, DC: National Academy of Sciences; 2011.
12. Centers for Disease Control and Prevention. The social-ecological model: a framework for prevention. Available at: http://www.cdc.gov/violenceprevention/overview/social-ecologicalmodel.html. Accessed July 22, 2016.
13. Ratts MJ, Singh AA, Nassar-McMillan S, et al. Multicultural and social justice counseling competencies. Available at: http://www.counseling.org/docs/default-source/competencies/multicultural-and-social-justice-counseling-competencies.pdf?sfvrsn=20. Accessed July 22, 2016.
14. Nadal KL, Skolnik A, Wong Y. Interpersonal and systemic microaggressions toward transgender people: implications for counseling. J LGBT Issues Couns 2012;6:55–82.
15. Peres WS. Structural violence and AIDS in the Brazilian transgender community. Revista de Psicologia da UNESP 2004;3(1):21–31.
16. Reisner SL, White Hughto JM, Gamarel KE, et al. Discriminatory experiences associated with posttraumatic stress disorder symptoms among transgender adults. J Couns Psychol 2016;63(5):509–19.
17. Lev AI, Alie L. Transgender and gender nonconforming children and youth: developing culturally competent systems of care. In: Fiser SK, Ponier JM, Blau GM, editors. Improving emotional and behavioral outcomes for LGBT youth: a guide for professionals. New York: Paul H. Brookes; 2012. p. 43–66.
18. Birkett M, Newcomb ME, Mustanski B. Does it get better? A longitudinal analysis of psychological distress and victimization in lesbian, gay, bisexual, transgender, and questioning youth. J Adolesc Health 2015;56(3):280–5.
19. Gay Lesbian Straight Educator's Network. The 2013 national school climate survey: the experiences of lesbian, gay, bisexual, and transgender youth in our nation's schools. 2013. Available at: http://www.glsen.org/nscs. Accessed July 22, 2016.
20. Huebner DM, Thoma BC, Neilands TB. School victimization and substance use among lesbian, gay, bisexual, and transgender adolescents. Prev Sci 2015; 16(5):734–43.
21. Singh AA, dickey lm. Introduction to trans-affirming counseling and psychological practice. In: Singh AA, dickey lm, editors. Affirmative counseling and psychological practice with transgender and gender nonconforming clients. Washington, DC: American Psychological Association; 2016. p. 3–18.
22. Singh AA, Burnes TR. Shifting the counselor role from gatekeeping to advocacy: ten strategies for using the ACA Competencies for Counseling with Transgender

Ellenis Intercounselling, practice, research and advocacy. J LGBT Issues Couns 2010;4:126–34.

23. Klonsky ED, Muehlenkamp JJ. Self-injury: a research review for the practitioner. J Clin Psychol 2007;63:1045–56.

24. Jacobson CM, Gould M. The epidemiology and phenomenology of non-suicidal self-injurious behavior among adolescents: a critical review of the literature. Arch Suicide Res 2007;11:129–47.

25. dickey lm, Reisner SL, Juntunen CL. Non-suicidal self-injury in a large online sample of transgender adults. Prof Psychol Res Pr 2015;46:3–11.

26. Henry JD, Crawford JR. The short-form version of the Depression Anxiety Stress Scales (DASS-21): construct validity and normative data in a large nonclinical sample. Br J Clin Psychol 2005;44:227–39.

27. Lovibond SH, Lovibond PF. Manual for the depression anxiety stress scales. Sydney (Australia): University of New South Wales; 1995.

28. Orbach I, Mikulincer M. The body investment scale: construction and validation of a body experience scale. Psychol Assess 1998;10(4):415–25.

29. Coleman E, Bockting W, Botzer M, et al. Standards of care for the health of transsexual, transgender, and gender nonconforming people, 7th version. Int J Transgend 2012;13:165–232.

30. Nock MK. Why do people hurt themselves? New insights into the nature and functions of self-injury. Curr Dir Psychol Sci 2009;18:8–83.

31. dickey lm. Non-suicidal self-injury in the transgender community (Order No. 3497800). Available from ProQuest Dissertation & Theses Global. (923848921). 2011.

32. Lev AI. Transgender emergence: therapeutic guide for working with gender variant people and their families. New York: Routledge; 2004.

33. Burnes TR, Dexter MM, Richmond K, et al. The experiences of transgender survivors of trauma who undergo social and medical transition. Traumatology 2016; 22(1):75–84.

34. American Psychological Association. Guidelines for psychological practice with transgender and gender nonconforming people. Am Psychol 2015;70(9):832–64.

35. Murad MH, Elamin MB, Garcia MZ, et al. Hormonal therapy and sex reassignment: a systemic review and meta-analysis of quality of life and psychosocial outcomes. Clin Endocrinol (Oxf) 2010;72:214–31.

# Affirmative Psychological Testing and Neurocognitive Assessment with Transgender Adults

Colton L. Keo-Meier, PhD[a,b,c],*, Kara M. Fitzgerald, PhD[d,1]

## KEYWORDS

- Affirmative • Transgender • LGBT • Assessment • Neuropsychology
- Neurocognitive • Testing

## KEY POINTS

- A level of competence above and beyond psychological assessment with the general population is necessary for an accurate and ethical interpretation of test data of transgender clients.
- An understanding of the gender-affirmative model (GAM) and the gender minority stress model should guide clinicians' choice of psychological tests, scoring, and interpretation and case conceptualization of transgender clients.
- Clinicians must attempt to distinguish mental health symptoms from clients' unique experiences of gender dysphoria.
- A medical decisional capacity model is in line with an affirmative assessment approach.

The history of assessment and psychological testing with transgender clients is fraught with challenges and barriers to accessing medically necessary gender transition–related care.[1] For decades, transgender people have been made to undergo psychological testing as a standard part of their attempts to access this care.[2] Even today, however, no consensus exists on best practices for assessment and psychological testing with transgender clients in general or in transgender-specific practice. As of this writing, no assessment instruments in neuropsychological, intelligence, or

The authors have nothing to disclose.
[a] Department of Psychology, University of Houston, Houston, TX 77204, USA; [b] School of Medicine, University of Texas Medical Branch, 301 University Boulevard, Galveston, TX 77555, USA; [c] Lee and Joe Jamail Specialty Care Center, Menninger Department of Psychiatry and Behavioral Sciences, Baylor College of Medicine, 1977 Butler Boulevard, Houston, TX 77030, USA; [d] Department of Psychology, Lemuel Shattuck Hospital, 170 Morton Street, Jamaica Plain, MA 02130, USA
[1] Present address: 158 Harvard Street #3, Brookline, MA 02446.
* Corresponding author. University of Texas Medical Branch, 301 University Boulevard, Galveston, TX 77555.
E-mail address: ckeo-meier@uh.edu

Psychiatr Clin N Am 40 (2017) 51–64
http://dx.doi.org/10.1016/j.psc.2016.10.011
0193-953X/17/© 2016 Elsevier Inc. All rights reserved.

personality testing batteries have been normed for validation for the transgender pop ulation. To further complicate matters, many tests have gender-based norms, leading to multiple questions, including which set of norms clinicians should use when assessing transgender clients—man or woman. Does it depend on if a client has started a medical transition? Does it even matter which gender is selected? Is it different depending on each instrument? Using the gender-affirmative model (GAM),[3] this article aims to answer these questions in the context of general clinical assessment and provide considerations for assessment and the use of psychological testing for evaluation for hormone therapy and surgery related to gender transition.

As the field of transgender health developed, decades of research have reported on data from psychological evaluations of transgender people. The findings from much of the early literature were based on results from the Minnesota Multiphasic Personality Inventory (MMPI) and other psychological tests.[4–6] The findings from this literature include high rates of psychopathology and mental health disparities in this population[7,8] and reports of transgender people and their partners having severe mental illness simply because they are transgender or for believing that their transgender partners are really the gender they say they are.[9] These interpretations were not informed by current theories, such as gender minority stress,[10] and fueled stigma and bias against transgender people in the mainstream. Furthermore, uninformed interpretations of many types of psychological tests have had devastating consequences to many transgender people, such as losing custody of their child and not being hired for a job.

Initial attempts to create standards of care by the World Professional Association for Transgender Health (WPATH) (then known as the Harry Benjamin International Gender Dysphoria Association), begun in the late 1970s, resulted in a gate-keeping model,[11] where transgender patients had to prove that they were transgender and pass the tests that clinicians instituted. Although there is a growing literature concerning assessment of gender dysphoria children,[12–14] there is no consensus among clinicians today regarding the role of psychological tests in evaluations for hormone and surgical treatment of gender transition in adults. It is becoming increasingly clear that both medical and surgical treatments are related to improved mental health outcomes in this marginalized group.[15–17] The practice of psychological testing using tests that are not normed on this population or for these purposes must be scrutinized.

## ESTABLISHING PROVIDER COMPETENCE

A level of competence above and beyond psychological assessment with the general population is necessary for an accurate and ethical interpretation of test data of transgender clients. Affirmative assessment with transgender clients stems from a clinician's understanding of transgender-affirming psychological practice.[1] Knowledge of the following is a prerequisite for transgender-affirmative assessment: the GAM,[3] the gender minority stress model,[10] the impact of hormone therapy on the mood and cognition of transgender people,[5,17–21] and considerations for scoring test data using gender-normed assessment instruments.

The GAM[3] informs assessment interpretation and case conceptualization with transgender clients. The major premises of this model inform the purposes of affirmative assessment. For example, the GAM posits that being transgender is not a disorder, gender diversity varies across cultures and requires cultural sensitivity, gender is not binary and may be fluid, and, if there is pathology, it is more likely formed in response to a hostile environment (transphobic and homophobic cultural reactions) than from within the person. The GAM defines gender health as the "opportunity to live in a gender that feels most real or comfortable"[3] to the person and to be able to express one's gender without being restricted or rejected. The American Psychological Association's guidelines on working with transgender clients also recommend an affirmative approach.[22]

Affirmative assessment is further informed by the gender minority stress model.[10] This model, informed by Meyer,[23] presents distal and proximal stressors experienced by this population, which has a negative impact on mental health. Distal stress factors include physical and sexual violence, harassment, and discrimination, all of which occur at a much higher rate in this population than in the general population.[7] Proximal stress factors include expectations of violence and internalized transphobia. These may appear to be symptoms of depression or paranoia. Mental health sequelae stemming from distal and proximal stressors include high rates of substance abuse and suicidal ideation and attempts consistent with a population dealing with significant experiences of trauma and rejection. A history of suicide attempts in this population has been established to be 10 to 20 times more likely than in the general population.[24] Community connectedness and a sense of trans in one's trans identity are resilience factors that are thought to buffer the effects of the stressors. The Gender Minority Stress and Resilience scale[25] assessment instrument has been developed to assess these specific factors and may assist in case conceptualization.

Another experience that is unique to the transgender population is that of gender dysphoria. According to the 7th version of the WPATH standards of care,[26] not all transgender people experience gender dysphoria; living in a society that is not welcoming or inviting of people whose gender identity is different from the sex assigned them at birth may lead to minority stressors, including traumatic experiences. Olson-Kennedy[27] asserts that transgender people may have multiple thoughts related to their gender, body, or physical safety on a daily basis. He refers to this experience as gender noise. For example, after shaving her face on a daily basis, resulting in skin abrasions and dryness, a trans woman may have recurring thoughts: "I wonder if people will know I'm trans. Will makeup even help me at this point? Is this whole process even worth it? Should I shave my face again? If I go on a date, will I ever come home again?" A trans boy in high school may spend so much energy dealing with gender noise that his academic performance may be significantly impacted. His gender noise may include thoughts, such as, "I wonder if I'll ever be able to start testosterone. Is my binder too tight? Can other people see my chest or is it flat enough? Why does my voice always give me away? Will anyone ever use my pronouns? Is my jawline masculine? Will I be able to hold my bladder so I don't have to try to use the bathroom at school?" It is possible that this unique thought process may not be apparent to the assessor who may be picking up on gender dysphoria yet conceptualizing it as inattention, lack of interpersonal interest, social anxiety, depression, and other psychological issues.

## DISTINGUISHING MENTAL HEALTH SYMPTOMS FROM GENDER DYSPHORIA

Because mental health disparities disproportionately have an impact on transgender persons,[8] affirmative assessors must attempt to parse out mental health symptoms from gender dysphoria.[22] If test results indicate a mental health condition, clinicians must consider possible explanations for this occurrence as it relates to a client's transgender history. The American Psychological Association guidelines[22] suggest several explanations, each of which is illustrated by cases developed for the purposes of this article.

Case 1: no relationship between the transgender history and the mental health condition. Example: a transgender man who has been on testosterone for 10 years has bipolar disorder that runs in his family. He is also trans but no longer experiences dysphoria related to his gender. He continues testosterone treatment to prevent symptoms of gender dysphoria and receives psychiatric and counseling services for his bipolar disorder.

Case 2: a gender concern leads to or exacerbates mental health symptoms directly through gender dysphoria and/or indirectly through gender minority stress, which may present as depression, anxiety, or paranoia. The gender concern itself does not cause the mental health condition. Examples: a nonbinary trans person has been chronically misgendered, has been rejected by several family members, and was fired from a job for not conforming to gender norms in the workplace; the experience of these gender minority stressors leads the client to develop symptoms consistent with social anxiety disorder. A transgender woman experiences severe gender dysphoria in the realm of genital dysphoria and is having difficulty concentrating in her college classes. A transgender boy develops an eating disorder as he is about to begin his endogenous puberty in efforts to delay menstruation. These last 2 examples demonstrate how the experience of gender dysphoria leads to mental health symptoms.

Case 3: the gender concern and mental health symptoms are independent, yet they influence each other, sometimes simultaneously. Neither actually causes the other. Examples: a transgender adult with a history of emotional dysregulation is about to begin hormone therapy and presents for therapy with a concern that the experience of a second puberty will have a negative impact on mood; a transgender man with an autism spectrum disorder speaks about his experience of gender in an uncommon manner and does not care if others see him as the man he knows himself to be.

Case 4: a mental health concern seems to be a gender concern, yet the real problem is not a true gender concern.[28] Example: a client states that they are a man living in woman's body and presents with psychotic symptoms. After the psychosis is treated, however, the client no longer expresses a gender concern. In these cases, the gender concern is a delusion, which occurs in the context of psychosis or mania and does not represent a true gender concern. This is an extremely rare presentation and should be assessed carefully.

In circumstances of gender dysphoria or transgender identity present (cases 1 and 3), treatment, including hormone therapy and/or surgical treatment, may be indicated.[26] Multiple professional organizations have published about the medical necessity and alleviating nature of these treatments in the transgender population.[29] In cases of gender dysphoria causing or exacerbating mental health symptoms (case 2), medical treatment of gender dysphoria is thought to be helpful in alleviating those symptoms as well.

## EFFECTS OF HORMONE THERAPY ON MOOD AND COGNITION

Because mood and cognition are factors considered in presurgical assessments, it is important to discuss the effects that hormone therapy has on these factors. There has been empirical evidence to suggest that there are differences between genders with respect to cognition in the cisgender (nontransgender) population. Namely, the data have supported similar overall IQ between genders while noting a divide between spatial and verbal intelligence. More specifically, women tend to have higher verbal intelligence, whereas men tend to have higher spatial intelligence.[30] The differences in spatial ability have been more robustly and consistently demonstrated.[31,32]

Given that hormonal findings have been posited, it stands to reason that cross-sex hormone administration is likely to have a bearing on cognition. Hormone therapy has been found to have an impact on mood and cognition in transgender adults, although research on cognition has yielded mixed results.[21] Several studies on hormone therapy have found associations with improved mental health, including increased quality of life,[33] decreased anxiety and depression,[16,18,34,35] decreased stress,[36,37] and decreased paranoia.[17] Among research that specifically examines the cognitive changes brought about by hormone therapy, a majority of studies have focused on spatial rotation and verbal fluency.[5,21] Increases in spatial ability have been the most robust findings related to testosterone therapy,[38] although some studies have not found significant improvement in spatial ability related to testosterone.[21] In 1 uncontrolled study,[38] trans men were shown to have increased scores on a measure of spatial rotation and decreases in verbal ability after 3 months on testosterone treatment. A later study, which used cisgender men or women as controls,[38] found similar results. A long-term follow-up study that used transgender women as controls was able to replicate spatial increases; however, findings indicated that verbal ability did not diminish in transgender men after over 1 year on testosterone.[39] A more recent study, however, was not able to replicate spatial gains in transgender men after 2.5 months on testosterone.[21] The latest longitudinal research on cognition in transgender men used a cross-sectional design to show improved performance on visual memory tasks relative to transgender men who were not on testosterone.[19] From this information, it seems likely that testosterone is related to increases in spatial skills; however, due to variable findings, testosterone's effect on verbal ability is less clear.

Furthermore, there have been structural differences noted even in pretransition populations, which may serve to confirm cognitive changes noted, although these findings have been mixed. Using diffusion tensor imaging, a type of imaging using water molecule tissue diffusion, which is effective at looking at axonal structures, Rametti and colleagues[40] noted that transgender men were significantly more similar to cisgender men than to cisgender women with respect to white matter microstructural pattern, in terms of axonal brain structure. Mood itself has been shown to have potential negative effects on cognition, in particular attention, which may serve to then affect cognition itself.[41–43] Thus, given that there are known effects of hormone therapy on mood,[16,17] there may be secondary effects of hormone therapy on cognitive functioning. These findings make a strong case for taking hormone status into consideration when interpreting findings, because of their potential effect test selection, normative data selection, and interpretation (discussed later).

## CONSIDERATIONS FOR GENERAL ASSESSMENT AND TESTING

The experience of gender dysphoria and being transgender in a cisgender world is incredibly profound. Being transgender has an impact on many different areas of psychological functioning in ways that leading researchers and clinicians are just beginning to elucidate. No formal guidelines exist for interpreting test data in light of the unique experiences of transgender client. Transgender clients may present for the same reasons that cisgender people present for psychological assessment. These include, but are not limited to, neuropsychological and personality testing. This section outlines specific considerations for these types of testing and discusses the use of instruments that rely on gender-based norms.

### Neuropsychological Assessment

Neuropsychological evaluations consist of batteries of standardized tests, which have been administered to large sets of individuals, ultimately creating a set of normative data. These data are often stratified by several factors, including age, education, race/ethnicity, and gender[44,45]; the last factor becomes a substantial point of consideration when conducting clinical evaluations of transgender individuals, particularly when considering the aforementioned evidence of cognitive changes with transition[31,32] as well as changes on imaging.

At this juncture, there does not exist a specific normative basis for transgender individuals. Furthermore, it is unlikely that such a normative basis will be on the horizon for the transgender population in the near future, for many if any tests, based on numerous much larger classes of minority individuals (eg, Asian Americans) have not yet been afforded this privilege. It has been established in many cases that minority individuals are often at a disadvantage, insofar as being overly pathologized when conventional normative data are used.[46,47] Thus, it seems unlikely that a comparatively smaller group of minority individuals, namely the transgender population, will be represented on a normative basis in the near future. The development of stratified normative data is further complicated because many transgender people represent multiple minority statuses. For example, norms for Hispanic lesbian transgender women will likely never exist.

Additionally, in the absence of specific normative data for this population, ideally research would be conducted to investigate which set of normative data to use. For example, in other such cases it has been determined that group X functions more closely overall to the Y set of norms and thus that can be adopted as a clinical standard to use, in the absence of group X's own set of normative data. With this dearth of transgender-specific normative data, it behooves the field to begin a discussion of best practices. Utilization of a test or task that does not use gender-stratified norms may be the optimal solution.

In the absence of tests normed on a transgender population, test selection should be a factor of consideration for clinicians. Many clinicians, however, may use fixed batteries or have measures that utilize gender-stratifed norms and with which they are more comfortable. Furthermore, there may exist good clinical reason to not use these measures in some occasions, for example, if there is not a measure of equal (to the clinician's standard measures) or acceptable (per the clinician's estimation) clinical rigor, whether with respect to the task itself, specific aspect of the domain assessed, or the robustness of the norms. Thus, in these cases, until the area has been better investigated, it may be most cautious and prudent to use a gender-stratified (ie, with normative data for both cisgender men and cisgender women) rigorous test, per the clinician's standards, with norms of the clinician's choosing based on clinical judgment and then proceed to score this with each set of gender norms. An additional step may then be to include a non–gender-normed measure within the same domain, such that comparisons can be made.

### Personality/Psychopathology Assessment

The most widely used personality instrument is the MMPI – 2nd edition (MMPI-2).[48] It is commonly used in evaluations that have an impact on personnel selection and custody hearings, areas where transgender people are typically discriminated against. MMPI-2 interpretations have significant implications for the lives of this population. Compared with controls, elevations have been reported on almost every scale in transgender samples.[6,17,49] MMPI-2 scales are designed to measure psychopathology (eg, hypochondria, depression, and paranoia). Scale elevations are interpreted as clinically significant and used to support diagnoses and inform treatment. Most reports indicate this population is more likely to show several scale elevations, especially the earlier they are in their identity development and transition process. This assessment tool has been used with transgender people for decades[50] and has been researched with this population more than any other personality assessment.[6,15,51] As such, the MMPI-2 is the focus of this section.

Cultural variables unique to the transgender population are thought to have an impact on the MMPI-2 scales and scales of similar personality assessment instruments. The hypochondria and hysteria scales may be influenced by experiences of gender dysphoria that revolve around bodily image disturbance. Depression and anxiety scales may be elevated as a result of gender minority stress, gender dysphoria, a combination of the 2, or independently. The psychopathic deviate scale is thought to be susceptible to elevations related to interpersonal difficulties caused by the overwhelming lack of acceptance of transgender people in society.[15] The masculinity/femininity scale may or may not be elevated depending on which gender template was used and if the person is gender conforming in gender expression. Elevations on the paranoia scale could be influenced by feelings of being misunderstood, mistreated, suspicious and guarded, lonely, resentful toward family members, and afraid of physical attack.[52] These paranoia scale elevations may be more of an indication of high rates of discrimination and family rejection[10,53,54] and thus may be realistic appraisals instead of a true measure of paranoia. Finally, increased scores on the schizophrenia scale may be reflective of strained family relationships, social alienation, and questioning of self-worth and identity.[48] Both paranoia and schizophrenia scales have also been found elevated in African American populations related to cultural mistrust and minority stress,[55] likely paralleling gender minority stress experienced in transgender populations.

Multiple MMPI-2 scores have been found to change in a more healthy direction after 3 months of hormone therapy in transgender men.[17] Previously, it had been well established that MMPI-2 profiles remain stable over the course of a lifetime.[56] Historically, transgender people were required or expected to undergo intensive psychotherapy as well as psychological testing before accessing hormone therapy. This finding of quick, positive shift in MMPI-2 scores was unexpected, because even intensive psychotherapy multiple times per week for a period of several years has not been found to have in impact on MMPI-2 scores.[57] Because this instrument is susceptible to significant changes related to hormone therapy to such an extent not previously been reported in the MMPI-2 literature,[17] it is not thought to present an accurate clinical picture of clients' psychological functioning present early in their gender transition.

Because the concepts of gender minority stress, gender dysphoria, and gender transition have only begun to be understood in the past few years, clinicians have been providing interpretations based on MMPI-2 data without considerations of how these concepts may be having an impact on the psychological functioning of their clients. Unfortunately, this lack of knowledge has likely harmed this population. For example, a transgender woman who is fighting for custody may have an MMPI-2 profile with elevations on scales 4 and 8. Traditionally, elevations on scales 4 and 8 are given a poor prognosis due to the characterological nature of the pattern of psychopathology.[52] Elevations in scales 4 and 8 in transgender clients, however, may not result from the same underlying psychological phenomena as in the general population. It is possible that scales 4 and 8 are elevated in this case because the scales are picking up on her experience of social ostracization, being fired from her job for being transgender (which is legal in her state), being removed from the restroom by police for not "looking like a woman," not being understood by her spouse who is divorcing her and attempting to take the children away from her because she is transgender, being chronically misgendered, and other common experiences shared by transgender individuals. Interpretation of her MMPI-2 scores without consideration of these variables is more likely to result in denying custody of her children than an affirmative (ie, competent) assessment. In this way, use of this test and other tests that are not normed on this population by clinicians who lack training with this population has resulted in harming an already vulnerable population. Due to susceptibility to change with hormone therapy, multiple unique cultural variables that must be brought into consideration, lack of normative data from the transgender population, and the potential for artificial scale elevations, MMPI-2 profiles should be used sparingly and interpreted with caution in this population, especially before initiation of medical or surgical transition.

### Do I Use the Men or Women Scoring Template?

The most common question asked by clinicians who are assessing transgender clients is, "Do I score them as man or woman?" There is no standardized method of choosing which template to use for transgender clients. Affirmative assessment should aim not to use any assessments that are scored based on cisgender gender norms, unless a nongendered scoring option does not exist. When faced with choosing a gender template, the question must first be pondered, "Is there a reason to use a gender-normed test with this client?" Ideally, clinicians would not use tests that are scored using gender (ie, cisgender) norms with this population, because those norms are more than likely created from all cisgender participants and are not generalizable to this population. It is most consistent with affirmative practice to use extensive history and symptom inventories to answer the assessment question if at all possible. If all these factors are considered and a gender-normed test still is used, it may be best to score using both templates. Because there are no norms for transgender clients on these tests, simply picking 1 template is not necessarily the most valid answer. Research has indicated that the choice of gender template may result in different findings,[17] so the choice does matter. Once the test is scored twice, it is advisable to interpret the findings in the context of the other data collected to determine if the findings from either the man or woman template are more in line with the rest of the information from the assessment. When writing up the results, be sure to indicate that tests were used that were not normed on this population, that results were generated using both gender templates, the rationale for relying more heavily on 1 gender template more than the other, and a statement the data should be interpreted with caution. If the template cannot be scored twice, using the gender of the template that is most congruent with the client's gender identity may feel affirming to clients who identify as either man or woman. Clinicians should be mindful that scoring with 1 gender template may result in higher levels of psychopathology than the other for the same test data, and this may have an impact with some scales more than others (MMPI-2).[17]

If using assessment inventories that have not been normed on this population may cause harm, what can be done to mitigate that harm? It is important to acknowledge that this problem exists and to recognize that many assessments fail to accurately represent the psychological functioning of transgender people and that interpretation of data without an affirmative, competent approach has caused harm to this population. One novel instrument, the Gender Minority Stress and Resilience scale,[25] may be used to generate data on a transgender person's experience of gender minority stress. Information gained from the Gender Minority Stress and Resilience scale could be used to inform more accurate case conceptualization when interpreting testing results from all other assessment instruments, because none currently exists that has been normed on this population. Until normative data with this population are created, clinicians should also consider not using standardized assessments and relying more heavily on the history in light of gender dysphoria, gender minority stress, and gender transition status. Scores of transgender clients may be artificially inflated and may not be indicative of psychopathology, especially if a client is early in the identity formation or gender transition process. The use of symptom inventories that do not use gender-based norms (eg, Beck Depression Inventory, 2nd edition, or Symptom

Checklist-90-Revised) may be considered as alternatives to the MMPI-2 and other measures of psychopathology. Typically, graduate-level assessment courses do not provide adequate training on testing with transgender clients. Therefore, continuing education as well as consultation with clinicians who have more knowledge and experience working with this population is an important step.

## EVALUATION FOR MEDICAL AND SURGICAL TRANSITION

/th version of the WPATH standards of care[26] provides criteria for hormone therapy and multiple surgeries related to gender transition. They also include guidance on domains of assessment, yet they do not mention specific psychological assessment inventories. This has led to individual practitioners creating their own assessment process, some including testing instruments whereas others relying on an extensive clinical interview with psychoeducation on effects and risks of the treatment. In this area, clinicians tend to work with limited evidence and without evidence-based assessment protocols. Those who are using assessment instruments to help answer the question of whether or not a client is ready for medical transition are using tools that were not created for the purposes they are used for. This is akin to attempting to screw on a lightbulb with a hammer. Taking the analogy a step further, deciding whether to use the female or male template is like deciding between a hammer with a larger striking face or a smaller striking face to screw on a lightbulb; neither is adequate or effective.

Given the dearth of literature or specific guidance with respect to evaluation for gender transition–related surgeries, to discuss best practice standards, it may be useful to examine these factors in other types of presurgical evaluations that are used in the general population. Evaluation protocols for epilepsy, organ transplant, and bariatric surgeries have a long history of research and practice.[58] When examining common themes in these types of evaluations, it is important to keep in mind that these evaluations do not, as a rule, involve only 1 minority population whose candidacy for evaluation is directly related to their minority status.

Presurgical evaluation of cognitive and mental health variables is common for various types of surgeries. The rationale behind requiring this type of evaluation or the reasoning for the best practice to include this, however, is variable given the risks involved to patients in the surgical procedure and purpose of the evaluation.[59] For example, when used for presurgical evaluations prior/to determine candidacy for epilepsy surgery, the goal has historically been to establish baseline level of cognitive functioning across domains and to predict postoperative performance, because there may be changes noted or expected in some cases. In the past, the purpose had historically included localizing zones of epileptogenic activity. This is no longer a focus of the evaluations, although they are still used to determine if there are widely discrepant findings between imaging and cognitive functioning (ie, if electrographic and cognitive data findings are not at in keeping).[60] These findings may ultimately determine appropriateness for surgery candidacy based on medical outcomes and help to track and predict cognitive outcomes.

In cases of transplant evaluations, wherein a donor organ is transplanted into a patient to replace a compromised organ, the goal is often to assess capacity for informed consent and willingness/capacity to adhere to appropriate aftercare, with the notion that this may have implications to the individual's overall health.[61] Although different guidelines exist depending on the type of transplant, each type of transplant assessment generally includes considerations of ability to adhere to after-care, quality of life, and likelihood of failure (from a medical standpoint).[62]

Conversely, the purpose of presurgical bariatric evaluations is different. For these evaluations, "[s]uccessful outcome for bariatric surgery is largely dependent on patients' ability to adhere to postoperative behavior changes,"[66] where successful outcome is weight reduction. This factor, success, has been found related to psychosocial and behavioral variables,[64,65] because there are interpersonal differences in adjusting to the modifications needed in lifestyle and eating behaviors that can be predicted to an extent by the aforementioned psychosocial and behavioral variables. Thus, this type of evaluation is aimed at determining whether or not the therapeutic intervention will be successful. As such, it has been argued that in this case a candidate should be "unconditionally" subjected to a psychological evaluation, not to deny surgical candidacy, but to "allow for early identification of factors potentially threatening the effectiveness of the treatment, but also for elimination or at least mitigation of their harmful influence on the surgical outcome."[64] As previously stated, it has been demonstrated that hormonal transition is more likely than extensive therapy to lead to positive MMPI-2 scores in transgender people; the transgender and bariatric surgery candidate populations and the relative purposes of presurgical evaluation differ fundamentally.[17]

In the bariatric surgery literature, there is a common belief that if clinically significant psychopathology symptoms are present and are related to current weight, they will resolve once weight loss has begun or postsurgically. This belief has not been consistently supported empirically, however, with some studies in support whereas other studies indicating persistence of symptoms postsurgically and still others indicating re-emergence of symptoms after initial resolution/abatement.[65] Were there a stronger relationship between resolution of symptoms of psychopathology that did mitigate or resolve after successful surgical outcome, it could be argued that there would be additional support to suggest that the presurgical evaluation should not be used in a gatekeeping manner.

In light of these apparent differences in the purpose and nature of presurgical evaluation for surgeries related to gender transition and those reviewed, a medical competency model may be best suited, in which individuals are evaluated for capacity to make medical decisions largely on their ability to understand risks and benefits of the procedure as well as alternatives, often in the form of an interview.[66,67] The functional elements of capacity can be broken into 4 elements,[66,68] namely, expressing choice (ie, the ability to communicate a treatment choice in a consistent manner without reflecting decisional impairment), understanding (ie, the ability to understand diagnostic and treatment information, including risks, benefits, and alternatives), appreciation (ie, ability to make meaning of how these consequences may play out in an individual's personal life), and reasoning (ie, ability to describe the aforementioned information in an individual's own terms and to process this information in a logical and rational manner).

These components are often best assessed through an interview, with the need for further testing only if 1 of these elements includes questions outside the scope of the interview or if questions about capacity remain after the interview is complete. Given the differences between presurgical evaluations with the transgender population and with presurgical evaluations for other populations, in addition to the notion that alternative forms of assessment are restrictive in nature, an interview based on the medical competency model would be the more affirmative and practice-supported form of presurgical evaluation. Although no standard clinical interview exists for presurgical evaluation in transgender clients, the use of psychological and neuropsychological assessment batteries are not included in an affirmative evaluation unless a specific case requires the collection of further information. An affirmative presurgical interview, at a minimum, includes a standard medical and mental health history, history of gender identity development, and preparedness for undergoing the specific procedure, including informed consent and education on preoperative and postoperative care as well as the procedure, social and family support, and practical preparation.[69]

## SUMMARY

As outlined in this article, standards for affirmative assessment with transgender clients are needed that are evidence based. The field is open for norming commonly used testing instruments as well as determining gender-neutral norms in tests that currently use a gender-based scoring and interpretation system. To avoid harm, clinicians who lack adequate knowledge and training on assessment with transgender clients should seek out supervision and consultation from more experienced clinicians and reach out to experts.

When conducting prehormone evaluations, assessors should keep in mind the evidence to support mood and cognitive changes associated with initiating hormone therapy. Although there is room for additional research exploring the mechanisms and predictors of such change, it cannot be presumed that no changes will occur after initiating hormone therapy. Furthermore, withholding hormone therapy from a transgender adult on the basis of suicidality or a mood disorder, which would likely respond well to hormone therapy, is not an affirmative practice and is likely to cause harm. Presurgical evaluations for surgery related to gender transition are fundamentally different from presurgical evaluations for other conditions in their purpose. A medical decisional capacity model is more in line with an affirmative assessment approach.

## REFERENCES

1. Singh A, dickey l. Introduction. Affirmative counseling and psychological practice with transgender and gender nonconforming clients. Washington, DC: Author; 2015.
2. Cohen-Kettenis P, Gooren L. Transsexualism: a review of etiology, diagnosis and treatment. J Psychosom Res 1999;46:315–33.
3. Hidalgo MA, Ehrensaft D, Tishelman AC, et al. The gender affirmative model: what we know and what we aim to learn. Hum Dev 2013;56:285–90.
4. Fleming M, Cohen D, Salt P, et al. A study of pre- and postsurgical transsexuals: MMPI characteristics. Arch Sex Behav 1981;10(2):161–70.
5. Gomez-Gil E, Vidal Hagomeijer A, Salamero M. MMPI-2 characteristics of transsexuals requesting sex reassignment: comparison of patients in prehormonal and presurgical phases. J Pers Assess 2008;90:368–74.
6. Miach P, Berah E, Butcher J, et al. Utility of the MMPI-2 in assessing gender dysphoric patients. J Pers Assess 2000;75:268–79.
7. Clements-Nolle K, Marx R, Katz M. Attempted suicide among transgender persons: the influence of gender-based discrimination and victimization. J Homosex 2006;51:50–69.
8. Hepp U, Kraemer B, Schnyder U, et al. Psychiatric comorbidity in gender identity disorder. J Psychosom Res 2005;58:259–61.
9. Fleming M, MacGowan B, Costos D. The dyadic adjustment of female-to-male transsexuals. Arch Sex Behav 1985;14:47–55.
10. Hendricks ML, Testa RJ. A conceptual framework for clinical work with transgender and gender nonconforming clients: an adaptation of the minority stress model. Prof Psychol Res Pract 2012;43:460–7.

11. Lev AI. Disordering gender: identity gender identity disorder in the DSM-IV-TR. J Psychol Human Sex 2005;17:35–69.

12. de Vries A, Cohen-Kettenis P. Management of gender dysphoria in children and adolescents: the Dutch approach. J Homosex 2012;59:301–20.

13. Edwards-Leeper L, Spack NP. Psychological evaluation and medical treatment of transgender youth in an interdisciplinary "Gender Management Service" (GeMS) in a major pediatric center. J Homosex 2012;59(3):321–36.

14. Leibowitz S, Telingator C. Assessing gender identity concerns in children and adolescents: evaluation, treatments, and outcomes. Curr Psychiatry Rep 2012; 14(2):111–20.

15. de Vries AL, Doreleijers TA, Steensma TD, et al. Psychiatric comorbidity in gender dysphoric adolescents. J Child Psychol Psychiatry 2011;52(11):1195–202.

16. Gómez-Gil E, Zubiaurre-Elorza L, Esteva I, et al. Hormone-treated transsexuals report less social distress, anxiety and depression. Psychoneuroendocrinology 2012;37:662–70.

17. Keo-Meier CL, Herman LI, Reisner SL, et al. Testosterone treatment and MMPI-2 improvement in transgender men: a prospective controlled study. J Consult Clin Psychol 2015;83(1):143–56.

18. Davis S, Meier SC. Effects of testosterone treatment and chest reconstruction surgery on mental health in female-to-male transgender people. Int J Sex Health 2014;26:113–28.

19. Gomez-Gil E, Canizares S, Torres A, et al. Androgen treatment effects on memory in female-to-male transsexuals. Psychoneuroendocrinology 2009;34:110–7.

20. van Goozen SHM, Cohen-Kettenis PT, Gooren LJG, et al. Activating effects of androgens on cognitive performance: causal evidence in a group of female-to-male transsexuals. Neuropsychologia 1994;32:1153–7.

21. van Goozen S, Slabbekoorn D, Gooren L, et al. Organizing and activating effects of sex hormones in homosexual transsexuals. Behav Neurosci 2002;116:982–8.

22. American Psychological Association. Guidelines for psychological practice with transgender and gender nonconforming people. Am Psychol 2015;70(9):832–64.

23. Meyer IH. Prejudice, social stress, and mental health in lesbian, gay, and bisexual populations: conceptual issues and research evidence. Psychol Bull 2003;129:674–97.

24. Blosnich J, Brown G, Shipherd J, et al. Prevalence of gender identity disorder and suicide risk among transgender veterans utilizing veterans health administration care. Am J Public Health 2013;103:e27–32.

25. Testa RJ, Habarth J, Peta J, et al. Development of the gender minority stress and resilience measure. Psychol Sex Orientat Gend Divers 2015;2(1):65–77.

26. Coleman E, Bockting W, Botzer M, et al. Standards of care for the health of transsexual, transgender, and gender-nonconforming people: version 7. Int J Transgend 2011;13:165–232.

27. Olson-Kennedy A. Clinical complexities of gender dysphoria. Presented at the annual Gender Infinity conference. Houston, TX, September 16, 2016.

28. Mizock L, Fleming M. Transgender and gender variant populations with mental illness: implications for clinical care. Prof Psychol Res Pract 2011;42(2):208–13.

29. Substance Abuse and Mental Health Services Administration. Ending conversion therapy: supporting and affirming LGBTQ youth. HHS Publication No. (SMA) 15–4928. Rockville (MD): Substance Abuse and Mental Health Services Administration; 2015.

30. Nowell A, Hedges LV. Trends in gender differences in academic achievement from 1960 to 1994: an analysis of differences in mean, variance and extreme scores. Sex Roles 1998;39:21–43.

31. Hyde J. The gender similarities hypothesis. Am Psychol 2005;60(6):581–92.

32. Wai J, Cacchio M, Putallaz M, et al. Sex differences in the right tail of cognitive abilities: a 30-year examination. Intelligence 2010;38:412–23.

33. Newfield E, Hart S, Dibble S, et al. Female-to-male transgender quality of life. Qual Life Res 2006;15:1447–57.

34. Colizzi M, Costa R, Todarello O. Transsexual patients' psychiatric comorbidity and positive effect of cross-sex hormonal treatment on mental health: results from a longitudinal study. Psychoneuroendocrinology 2014;39:65–73.

35. Danovitch P, Lundin PA, Murphy KJ. The evaluation of renal transplant candidates: clinical practice guidelines1. Cancer 1995;8:11.

36. Dubois LZ. Associations between transition-specific stress experience, nocturnal decline in ambulatory blood pressure, and C-reactive protein levels among transgender men. Am J Hum Biol 2012;24:52–61.

37. Meier SC, Fitzgerald K, Pardo S, et al. The effects of hormonal gender affirmation treatment on mental health in female- to-male transsexuals. J Gay Lesb Ment Health 2011;15:281–99.

38. van Goozen S, Cohen-Kettenis P, Gooren L, et al. Gender differences in behaviour: activating effects of cross-sex hormones. Psychoneuroendocrinology 1995;20:343–63.

39. Slabbekoorn D, van Goozen S, Megens J, et al. Activating effects of cross-sex hormones on cognitive functioning: a study of short-term and long-term hormone effects in transsexuals. Psychoneuroendocrinology 1999;24:423–47.

40. Rametti G, Carrillo B, Gomez-Gil E, et al. The microstructure of white matter in male to female transsexuals before cross-sex hormonal treatment. A DTI study. J Psychiatr Res 2011;45:949–54.

41. Elliott R. The neuropsychological profile in unipolar depression. Trends Cogn Sci 1998;2:447–54.

42. Porter RJ, Robinson LJ, Malhi GS, et al. The neurocognitive profile of mood disorders–a review of the evidence and methodological issues. Bipolar Disord 2015;17:21–40.

43. Rametti G, Carrillo B, Gomez-Gil E, et al. White matter microstructure in female to male transsexuals before cross-sex hormonal treatment. A diffusion tensor imaging study. Psychoneuroendocrinology 2012;37:1261–9.

44. Mitrushina M, Boone KB, Razani J, et al. Handbook of normative data for neuropsychological assessment. New York: Oxford University Press; 2005.

45. Strauss E, Sherman EM, Spreen O. A compendium of neuropsychological tests: administration, norms, and commentary. American Chemical Society; 2006.

46. Campbell AL Jr, Ocampo C, Rorie KD, et al. Caveats in the neuropsychological assessment of African Americans. J Natl Med Assoc 2002;94(7):591.

47. Heaton RK, Taylor M, Manly J. Demographic effects and use of demographically corrected norms with the WAIS-III and WMS-III. Clinical Interpretation of the WAIS-III and WMS-III 2003;181.

48. Butcher J, Graham J, Tellegen A, et al. Minnesota multiphasic personality inventory—2 (MMPI-2): manual for administration, scoring, and interpretation (Rev. Ed.). Minneapolis (MN): University of Minnesota Press; 2001.

49. de Vries A, Kreukels B, Steensma T, et al. Comparing adult and adolescent transsexuals: an MMPI-2 and MMPI-A study. Psychiatry Res 2011;186:414–8.

50. Leavitt F, Berger J, Hoeppner J, et al. Presurgical adjustment in male transsexuals with and without hormonal treatment. J Nerv Ment Dis 1980;168(11):693–7.
51. Tsushima W, Wedding D. MMPI results of male candidates for transsexual surgery. J Pers Assess 1979;43(4):385–7.
52. Duckworth J, Anderson W. MMPI & MMPI–2 interpretation manual for counselors and clinicians. 4th edition. Levittown (PA): Taylor & Francis; 1995.
53. Bockting WO, Miner MH, Swinburne Romine RE, et al. Stigma, mental health, and resilience in an online sample of the US transgender population. Am J Public Health 2013;103:943–51.
54. Lombardi E, Wilchins RA, Priesing D, et al. Gender violence: transgender experiences with violence and discrimination. J Homosex 2002;42:89–101.
55. Frueh BC, Smith DW, Libet JM. Racial differences on psychological measures in combat veterans seeking treatment for PTSD. J Pers Assess 1996;66:41–53.
56. Spiro A, Butcher JN, Levenson RM, et al. Change and stability in personality: a 5-year study of the MMPI-2 in older men. In: Butcher JN, editor. Fundamentals of MMPI-2: research and application. Minneapolis (MN): University of Minnesota Press; 2000. p. 443–62.
57. Gordon RM. MMPI/MMPI-2 changes in long-term psychoanalytic psychotherapy. Issues Psychoanal Psychol 2001;23:59–79.
58. Mitchell K. Preoperative evaluation. Am Fam Physician 2000;62(2):387–96.
59. King M. Preoperative evaluation. Am Fam Physician 2000;62:387–96. Northwestern University Medical School, Chicago (IL).
60. Rosenow F, Lüders H. Presurgical evaluation of epilepsy. Brain 2001;124:1683–700.
61. Danovitch GM, Cohen DJ, Weir MR, et al. Current status of kidney and pancreas transplantation in the United States, 1994–2003. American Journal of Transplantation 2005;5:904–15.
62. Steinman TI, Becker BN, Frost AE, et al. Guidelines for the referral and management of patients eligible for solid organ transplantation. Transplantation 2001; 71(9):1189–204.
63. Bauchowitz AU, Gonder-Frederick LA, Olbrisch ME, et al. Psychosocial evaluation of bariatric surgery candidates: a survey of present practices. Psychosom Med 2005;67(5):825–32.
64. Dziurowicz-Kozlowska AH, Wierzbicki Z, Lisik W, et al. The objective of psychological evaluation in the process of qualifying candidates for bariatric surgery. Obes Surg 2006;16:196–202.
65. Edwards-Hampton SA, Wedin S. Preoperative psychological assessment of patients seeking weight-loss surgery: identifying challenges and solutions. Psychol Res Behav Manag 2015;8:263–72.
66. American Bar Association, & American Psychological Association. Assessment of older adults with diminished capacity: a handbook for psychologists. Washington, DC: Author; 2008.
67. Sabatino CP. The new uniform health care decisions act: paving a health care decisions superhighway? MD Law Rev 1994;53:1238.
68. Berg JW, Appelbaum PS, Lidz CW, et al. Informed consent: legal theory and clinical practice. New York: Oxford University Press; 2001.
69. Deutsch M. Gender- affirming surgeries in the era of insurance coverage: developing a framework for psychosocial support and care navigation in the perioperative period. J Health Care Poor Underserved 2015;27:1–6.

# Barriers, Challenges, and Decision-Making in the Letter Writing Process for Gender Transition

Stephanie L. Budge, PhD[a],*, lore m. dickey, PhD[b]

## KEYWORDS

- Transgender • Gender diverse • Letter writing • Transition • Barriers
- Decision-making

## KEY POINTS

- Clinicians must advocate on behalf of their transgender and gender diverse (TGD) clients.
- Clinicians must use culturally appropriate and sensitive approaches in their work with TGD clients.
- Challenging clinical situations do not automatically lead to a lack of support for medical transition.
- Clinicians are encouraged to adopt an informed consent model when working with transitioning clients.
- Complex clinical situations (eg, co-occurring disorders) do not constitute contraindications to transition; rather they highlight the importance of consultation and collaboration.

## STANDARDS OF CARE

In 2011, the World Professional Association for Transgender Health (WPATH) provided the most recent version of the Standards of Care (SOC) version (v.) 7[1] Though there continue to be criticisms and need for revisions of the current SOC, the seventh version is generally considered less stigmatizing than the previous editions. In the current SOC, a letter from a mental health or medical provider is recommended for hormone therapy or chest surgery, and 2 letters are recommended for genital surgeries.[2,3] Although letters are not technically required, the WPATH SOC are considered the

Disclosure Statement: Neither author has a conflict of interest nor are we receiving any funding for this work.
[a] University of Wisconsin-Madison, 1000 Bascom Mall, 309 Education Building, Madison, WI 53706, USA; [b] Northern Arizona Univeristy, 801 South Knoles Drive, PO Box 5774, Flagstaff, AZ 86011-5774, USA
* Corresponding author.
E-mail address: budge@wisc.edu

primary standards worldwide and meet insurance companies (if they cover trans health care) will not cover the surgeries without these letters, and most surgeons will not accept a client without this documentation. Within the United States, there is a small faction of health care providers who use the informed consent model and, instead of requiring letters for medical interventions, will conduct a general assessment to determine if the individual can provide informed consent about the procedures.[4]

## THE GATEKEEPING ROLE

A large body of scholarship elucidates factors that contributed to understanding why mental health providers and physicians were regulated to the role of gatekeepers in the gender transition process.[1,5,6] The major focus of this literature is the historical factors that led to the stigmatization of transgender and gender diverse (TGD) persons within mental health and medical communities, as well as the experience of bias, prejudice, and discrimination in society as a whole.[7,8] Although consensus exists that TGD persons are highly stigmatized, disagreement persists as to why this bias continues. Several theorists indicate that a large portion of the population is doubtful about the realness of TGD identities.[9,10] TGD identity is assumed to be a phase; thereby lending support to the existence of transgender regret.[11]

One of the criticisms of the gatekeeping process of TGD individuals includes the concept that any individual can engage in body alterations (from plastic surgery to augmenting body parts) without gatekeeping. However, this argument does not withstand the notion that TGD individuals receive hormones and surgery because it is considered medically necessary care, whereas modification for other reasons is not considered medically necessary.[12] Based on the notion of the medical interventions being medically necessary, gender transition surgeons and insurance companies have turned to other health professionals to ensure that the client is psychologically healthy enough to consent to the process. Similar to TGD clients, individuals seeking bariatric surgery are also required to undergo psychological evaluations for readiness for medical interventions. Due to a lack of professional consensus around clinical decision-making and psychological evaluations for TGD clients, researchers and clinicians argue these concerns also exist for practitioners working with clients seeking bariatric surgeries.[13]

## ASSESSMENT OF PSYCHOLOGICAL HEALTH

The determination of whether or not a TGD individual is psychologically healthy enough for medically related gender transition procedures is unclear. First, there is no scientific consensus of what it means for a TGD (or a cisgender) individual to be psychologically healthy. According to the SOC, the clinician writing the letter has the responsibility to deem the client fit for medical intervention.[1] Even though the most updated SOC were released in 2011, there continues to be controversy from an understanding of psychological health from SOC v.6 to v.7. The SOC v.6[14] states, "the presence of psychiatric co-morbidities does not necessarily preclude hormonal or surgical treatment, but some diagnoses pose difficult treatment dilemmas and may delay or preclude the use of either treatment." Whereas the wording in the most up-to-date version indicates, "The presence of co-existing mental health concerns does not necessarily preclude possible changes in gender role or access to feminizing/masculinizing hormones or surgery; rather, these concerns need to be optimally managed prior to or concurrent with treatment of gender dysphoria."[1] Although neither of these statements indicates that co-occurring psychiatric disorders do not constitute grounds for denial of clinicians' support, the wording from the SOC v.6 was used to preclude many individuals from gaining access to medical interventions.[15–17] TGD individuals are advised by others in the transgender community to downplay any symptoms of anxiety, depression, and suicidality in case these might be used by clinicians as justification for exclusion and/or delay of treatment. The SOC v.7 have attempted to remedy this issue because research has shown that gender-specific medical interventions alleviate psychological distress.[18] Despite a cultural shift in understanding what psychologically healthy means, clients remain unsure of how honest they can be within psychological assessments for letters due to longstanding mistrust of mental health clinicians among members of the TGC community.[8,19,20]

## LETTER WRITING GUIDELINES

Evidence-based psychological practice with TGD clients remains in its infancy. Therefore, most clinicians who are considered qualified under the SOC, are operating within their understanding of best practices. Due to the lack of empirically supported guidelines regarding appropriate assessments and clinical decision-making for TGD clients, clinicians writing letters often find themselves at odds with how to handle complex clinical cases. Currently, clinicians are directed to seek consultation for particularly complex cases. Even those who offer consultation do so by relying on anecdotal experience rather than empirically supported practice guidelines.

Before 2015, almost no published papers were written to provide specific guidelines for writing letters for TGD clients. Within the last year, 2 publications have been written to provide clinicians with guidance in the letter writing process (Ducheny and colleageues, unpublished data, 2016).[21] Budge's[21] evidence-based case study detailed the assessment and, specifically, the psychological impact of letter writing in the treatment of a young adult TGD client. Results from the Center for Epidemiologic Studies Depression Scale (short form),[22] the Schwartz Outcome Scale,[23] the K10-Self-Administered Questionnaire,[24] and the Client Task Specific Change Measure-Revised[25] indicated that the client's quantitative measures of mental health improved immediately after she received her letter. The client reported feeling validated by seeing her chosen name and female pronouns written in a document about her; conversely, she also reported feeling both distress and anger in response the requirement that a gender dysphoria (GD) diagnosis be provided. Ducheny and colleagues (unpublished data, 2016) provide guidelines for writing letters and include several appendices with sample hormone, surgery, K-12 school, safe passage, and name change letters. There are also several additional resources available about how to conduct clinical assessments for the letter writing process. However, it is important to note that the pace of change is rapid and language and TGD-focused practices quickly become outdated.[26–31]

## CLINICAL DECISION-MAKING AND CULTURAL COMPETENCE

Although more resources are becoming available, such as competency standards within professions, transgender health is still relatively new.[5,32] Few medical or psychological practices are evidence-based as a direct result of a lack of attention paid to TGD clients. Part of the reason why specific mental health evidence-based practices may not yet exist for clinicians may be due to the lack of graduate training and clinicians not feeling competent to work with transgender individuals. Clinicians across all health care fields report this lack of competence. Sixty percent of endocrinologists rate themselves as "a little" to "not at all" competent to work with transgender patients, and 58% of the endocrinologists indicate "a little less" and "much less comfort in working with transgender patients.[38] Clients who have received mental health treatment report that many of the therapists they have seen have not been competent to work with them on gender-related issues.[19,34–36] Sixty-six percent of social workers indicate that they have "no knowledge" to "minimal knowledge" of transgender issues, and 68% of social workers indicate having "no competence" to "minimal competence."[37] In psychiatry, researchers have found that cisgender female psychiatrists report more positive attitudes than cisgender male psychiatrists.[38] Research in psychology[39] and counseling repeat the finding of cisgender male therapists having more negative attitudes than cisgender female therapists.[40] It is hypothesized that cisgender men display more prejudice toward TGD people because they are more invested in adhering to gender norms than cisgender women as a means to ensuring that their masculinity is upheld.[41]

Given the lack of perceived competence from both the practitioners and clients, and the lack of evidence-based practice, clinicians often find themselves feeling unsure of making decisions about how to proceed with complex cases. Little attention has been paid to how clinicians approach decisions regarding letter writing in complex clinical situations. The field is primarily focused on how to write letters rather than the impact of these letters. As well, there are few to no guidelines if complex clinical situations arise that lead to a clinician being unsure about whether or not they should write the letter. The medical field is much more advanced with research focused on clinical decision-making and clinical errors. In mental health fields, general information related to making errors in clinical judgment or clinical decision-making is sparse. A recent meta-analysis on clinical decision-making indicates that therapist confidence contributes to a small effect in predicting the accuracy of clinical decision-making, such that when clinicians feel more confident, they make more accurate decisions.[42] Because confidence related to comfort and competence seems to be low across the board, it is likely that clinical decision-making affects TGD mental health and treatment.

The purpose of this article is to elucidate some of the frequently encountered clinical issues and challenges associated with TGD clients who are interested in transitioning. The authors present an amalgam of cases that have occurred within our clinical practices to provide context for challenges and barriers that can occur within the context of clinical decision-making for letter writing. Most clinical cases are not clear-cut. The following 3 case examples were thematically chosen to highlight the primary areas in which clinicians experience challenging decision-making: (1) systemic issues, (2) interdisciplinary management of care, and (3) co-occurring mental health concerns.

## CHALLENGE ONE: SYSTEMIC CONCERNS

Many activists, practitioners, and scholars have criticized systemic oppression toward TGD individuals within the health care system.[20] These criticisms include institutional discrimination, such as a lack of insurance coverage,[43] provider discrimination,[44] and access to care.[45]

The GD diagnosis is a way in which systemic oppression can occur within the letter writing process for TGD clients. Many scholars indicate that this diagnosis is pathologizing.[17,46–50] In the most recent version of the *Diagnostic and Statistical Manual of Mental Disorders* (DSM)-5[51] the committee tasked with revising the gender identity diagnosis (GID) from the DSM-IV-TR[52] indicated that a primary reason to maintain a psychiatric diagnosis was to provide a code indicating medical necessity for hormone and surgical treatments.[53] Lev[17] argues that the psychiatric diagnosis is not necessary given that medical codes can exist for medical treatments that are not considered pathology (eg, pregnancy).

I (SB) have struggled with the challenges of providing a GD diagnosis when writing letters for TGD clients. In my clinical experience, most doctors requesting letters for hormones or surgery require a GID or GD diagnosis (depending on if they use the *International Classification of Diseases* 10th revision or DSM-5 criteria). It has always been my personal standpoint that having a transgender, gender nonconforming, or gender diverse identity does not constitute having a disorder. The current SOC[1] address this issue.

A disorder is a description of something with which a person might struggle, not a description of the person or the person's identity. Thus, transsexual, transgender, and gender nonconforming individuals are not inherently disordered.

I disagree with the SOC standpoint that giving a GD diagnosis is not the same as indicating that transgender identity is disordered. When writing letters for a TGD client, I, like almost all gender therapists, provide a GD diagnosis only in cases in which this is considered a requirement of medical providers. In their survey of gender therapists, Whitehead and colleagues[7] reported that 94% of their respondents indicated that they provided a GD diagnoses with reluctance and many were outspoken in their rejection of this diagnosis.

In a previous article, I outlined the case of Lia,[a] an 18 year-old Latina-Italian trans woman.[21] Lia provided informed consent for me to report the psychological outcomes of our therapeutic process and the impact of letter writing on her psychological health. Overall, her psychological outcomes improved because of her access to, and receipt of, hormone therapy; however, she indicated that she felt angry, sad, and upset that I was required to give her a GD diagnosis. I had numerous conversations about giving a GD diagnosis to clients; it is a rare case when clients feel neutral about the diagnosis. Usually, clients are compliant and indicate that they understand it is a necessary part of the process. They often follow this up with reporting some disappointment, anger, shame, or sadness around the diagnosis. When clients report such negative responses to being given the diagnosis of GD, I find myself unduly challenged. My job is to support clients and help them navigate their lives. Sometimes this means that I give feedback that clients may not like or that they find difficult to incorporate. However, the feedback is always clinically indicated and rooted in theory and evidence. When I provide a GD diagnosis, it is only because it is required and not because it is rooted in theory and evidence.

There are several ways I have learned to navigate the process of writing letters and providing a diagnosis. Because I have observed that it is often harmful to provide a GD diagnosis, I take steps to determine if the diagnosis is absolutely necessary. This means contacting providers who request letters and determining their reasoning for wanting the GD diagnosis and seeing if other options are available. I have had some success in this regard. However, my clinical experience has been that most providers will maintain the requirement. All providers have found it sufficient when I have worded my letters indicating that my client "meets criteria for GD" and outlining the specific criteria, rather than indicating that I am diagnosing the client with GD.

If it is determined that a GD diagnosis is a requirement of medical providers, I first ask clients about their thoughts and feelings about this diagnosis. If the diagnosis does not cause much distress for the client, it is likely that this conversation will be short. However, in my experience, clients want to process their thoughts and feelings

---

[a] NOTE: All client presentations in this article use pseudonyms for clients and providers. In addition to de-identifying the cases; these cases represent a compilation of clinical concerns from our respective work.

of and the diagnosis and what it means for the therapeutic relationship for the clinician to give this diagnosis. After listening to the client's reactions to the diagnosis, I offer my own relationship to the diagnosis and talk with the client about how and why I am wording the GD diagnosis in the letter. Clients often feel relieved to have the conversation about the diagnosis spoken out loud and I have noticed that this improves the therapeutic relationship.

## CHALLENGE TWO: MANAGEMENT OF CARE

Although it is a good clinical skill to learn how to work within interdisciplinary health care teams, many individuals are not trained to work within interdisciplinary teams or to consult across disciplines.[54] Schmaling and colleagues[55] provide information related to the positive impact of clinical trainees learning how to consult with an interdisciplinary team; specifically, that it is useful to learn different viewpoints of clinical situations to understand multiple ways to engage in decision-making. Dewey[3] conducted a qualitative study related to collaborative care between medical doctors and mental health professionals who work with shared TGD clients. Several treatment dilemmas were discussed, including lack of preservice knowledge, lack of supportive policies by employers and health care systems, inconsistent or inaccurate treatment documents, and reliance on clients to educate the providers.

Early in my (SB) professional career, I was given a training opportunity to work with an interdisciplinary collaborative care team that comprised a psychiatrist, nurse, social worker, psychologist, and occupational therapist in an inpatient hospital setting. This experience afforded me with the unique opportunity to consult and collaborate with surgeons and specialists who prescribed hormones to TGD clients. Later, in my capacity as a consultant to clinicians, I discovered that most therapists are unaccustomed to working in an interdisciplinary collaborative milieu.

To illustrate a specific challenging situation with managing collaborative care, I provide the case of Alex, a 24-year-old genderqueer individual. Sairah, a psychiatrist in the community where I was working at the time, had contacted me because she had been seeing Alex for a year every 3 weeks to conduct psychotherapy and medication management; she had obtained a release of information to consult with me about Alex. She had indicated that she had never worked with a transgender or genderqueer client and said that she was particularly worried about her competency to work with Alex. Sairah had indicated to me that Alex wanted to have chest masculinization surgery and that she was worried about supporting this for 2 reasons: (1) Alex was not reporting an interest in identifying as a man or using testosterone and (2) Alex had a family history of schizophrenia.

Several challenges occurred after this initial consultation. First, when Sairah started talking about Alex, she was using she, her, and hers pronouns for Alex. When I asked Sairah what pronouns Alex was using, she said that Alex preferred gender neutral pronouns (they, them, and theirs) but that she thought that it was too hard to use them and did not think it was necessary. This was a great teaching moment to talk with Sairah about using gender neutral pronouns and how she might be able to use them with her client to show her support of Alex's identity. I used gentle confrontation and education to talk with Sairah about the pronouns ("Yes, sometimes it can be difficult to learn how to use new pronouns. I find that my clients experience less distress when I use the pronoun that is fitting for them. I usually practice using gender neutral pronouns in my daily life so I can get used to what it is like with clients.") She was dismissive of this intervention and seemed to want to move on to get information about the 2 concerns previously listed.

I indicated to her that clients are not required to have any specific order or way of transitioning, meaning that some clients feel that they need surgery and not hormones, some clients feel they need hormones and not surgery, and some clients do not feel that they need either. Sairah seemed to respond well to this information. We discussed how she might be able to talk with her client about figuring out what her client's needs were for gender transitioning. Next, we discussed her concern about a family history of schizophrenia. She was particularly worried that her client's desire for chest masculinization surgery was a manifestation of the beginning of a psychotic disorder. We discussed other ways in which her client had exhibited symptoms of psychosis. She indicated that, other than having blunted affect, her client did not exhibit any other symptoms. I agreed to see Alex for a psychological evaluation to rule out psychosis but also indicated to Sairah that even if Alex was exhibiting beginning signs of having a psychotic disorder that would not necessarily preclude Alex from receiving gender-affirming care. Instead, it would require more consultation about how the co-occurring disorders were affecting each other.

I met Alex and Alex's father, Jordan, (whom Alex lived with and was very supportive) for several assessment sessions. After meeting with Alex and conducting a clinical interview, I determined that Alex did not seem to be exhibiting any signs of psychosis. However, Sairah had discussed with Alex and Jordan that she was concerned about Alex having a psychotic disorder and thus they expressed this concern with me and asked me to do a full psychological battery. I talked with Sairah about the pros and cons of conducting the psychological battery. First, we discussed her reasoning behind sharing her concerns about Alex having a psychotic disorder when there was no evidence to support this. She had concluded that she had wished she had not shared this information with the family. Alex and Jordan indicated that they thought it would be therapeutic for Alex to complete the psychological assessments to provide some reassurance to Alex that they were not experiencing psychotic symptoms, thus we decided to complete the battery. The results of the assessment were as expected and the battery provided Sairah with important clinical information to work through some traumatic issues from the past.

The battery also provided Sairah and me a platform to discuss Alex from the same clinical standpoint. When Sairah and I had initially consulted, she was the only one with any clinical information and I was providing my opinion without actually knowing Alex. We were able to collaborate about helping Sairah affirm Alex's identity and to better conceptualize Alex's presenting concerns. We decided that we would write a letter together for Alex's chest masculinization surgery. Throughout our consultation, Sairah seemed to become less reluctant to use gender neutral pronouns. Our collaboration had offered opportunities for me to model using they, them, or their pronouns for Alex and writing up the psychological battery provided an example of a written document that used Alex's gender neutral pronouns. As part of our consultation, we decided that I would provide Sairah with a general outline of how to write a letter and what she may want to provide in Alex's case but that she would write the letter to practice using Alex's pronouns and to gain experience in writing the letter. We also jointly contacted the surgeon to discuss what he wanted included in the letter and how we would want to portray our work with Alex.

I provide this example to show that consultations can be collaborative and ultimately lead to psychoeducation for the provider and for the client. I commend providers who consult about client concerns. It is easy for providers to pretend they have competence and provide incompetent care to a client, or alternately providers may simply refer the client to another practitioner to avoid consultation and further training. Although there were a few missteps throughout the example provided, ultimately, Alex reported that they felt relieved about the results from the psychological battery and they were able to obtain chest masculinization surgery. Their psychological outcomes after surgery had greatly improved. As well, the outcomes for Sarah were such that she was more comfortable using gender neutral pronouns, had a greater understanding of the individual ways TGD clients transition, and a clearer understanding of how she pathologized gender incongruence (thinking it was a psychotic symptom). She was also able to obtain practice writing letters and felt more comfortable consulting and collaborating with me after our work with Alex.

I also provide this example because I generally find consulting with other providers to be a positive experience. There are 2 factors that assisted with my comfort in seeking out consultation: (1) I had specific training working on interdisciplinary teams who consulted on a daily basis when I was a graduate student and (2) early in my private practice, I made a clinical error that would have been prevented if I had consulted about a case. This experience humbled and motivated me to seek consultation regularly.

I needed quite a bit of consultation when I first started working with TGD clients and I believe it is essential for more providers to be competent in their care with TGD clients. On a fairly regular basis, I find myself correcting pronouns and names for clients with the providers who contact me. Although it may seem benign to the provider, these mistakes are often reported to me as feeling highly dismissive and hurtful to clients. I recommend that if and when a provider makes a mistake related to their clients' pronouns, they should determine if they are reacting defensively when being corrected and where the defensive reaction is coming from. I recommend that providers practice using different pronouns in their daily lives so that they can get used to the process. I also recommend that providers take detailed notes with the client's pronouns so that they can make the cognitive connection of the pronoun with the client.

## CHALLENGE THREE: CO-OCCURRING MENTAL HEALTH CONCERNS

This case example focuses on the common types of clinical concerns that may be a contraindication to the commencement of a medical transition. The focus here is on some challenging mental health concerns that may be present for gender diverse clients.

One of the tasks of mental health professionals is to "assess, diagnose, and discuss treatment options for coexisting mental health concerns."[1] Gender diverse people seek mental health care for a wide variety of reasons and, in some cases, this has little or nothing to do with the client's gender identity. The mental health concerns exhibited by gender diverse people include a wide variety of diagnostic concerns. These concerns may include depression, anxiety, substance abuse, and autism spectrum disorders.[32,56,57] The WPATH SOC state that co-occurring mental health concerns should be "reasonably well-controlled."[1] The challenge is, however, that there is no clear indication of what well-controlled looks like in a clinical setting.

### The Case of Beatrice

Beatrice is a 23-year-old female-identified person referred to counseling by her primary care provider (Dr Terry Mason) for a clinical assessment and referral for hormone treatment. Beatrice came to my (lmd) office seeking hormone treatment after a long history of gender concerns. Her primary care physician was generally supportive of TGD clients but in Beatrice's case the physician had expressed concern about Beatrice's history of suicidal ideation, cutting, substance abuse, and a lack of basic personal hygiene. Beatrice reported being clean and sober for 63 days. She had recently been discharged from her second treatment facility. The first time she was in treatment for 90 days and she was able to maintain her sobriety for an additional 44 days.

Beatrice reported that she often felt quite distressed when going out in public. When she presented in male attire, which happened infrequently, people were hostile toward her yelling "faggot!" and "faerie!" and other homonegative statements. When she presented in female attire she felt as though she "had to defend herself from repeated unwanted sexual advances." To cope with this and other stressors she often engaged in self-injury, specifically cutting. She stated that "cutting helps me cope with the emotional difficulties" and "when I cut myself I feel disconnected from my troubles." Beatrice began cutting at the age of 14 years. She hid this behavior from her family and was relieved on beginning college when she found that several of her close friends also engaged in cutting. This helped her to feel more normal. Beatrice reported that sometimes drinking and using drugs (marijuana) have helped "calm my nerves."

Beatrice had never been in counseling for her gender concerns. She was reluctant to share and tended to be a poor historian. Beatrice had not told her family about her plans to medically transition (hormones only) or about her visits to counseling. I (lmd) shared some of the physician's concerns about Beatrice because I found it difficult to relate with Beatrice and I was unsure how to proceed in my work.

As I deepened my clinical relationship with Beatrice, it became apparent that she did not engage in basic personal hygiene. When I queried her about this, she stated that "I have too much distress about my body to take a shower." It also became apparent that Beatrice relied on her parents for a significant amount of financial support. In some ways, it seemed that Beatrice was not an independent adult. Similar to Dr Mason, I was beginning to have questions about whether Beatrice was ready to initiate hormone treatment.

Beatrice asked in session if I would contact her parents to ask for their support. She stated that she had told them of her plans and they were not supportive. We agreed to hold a joint session with her parents. During this session, her parents stated that this was "simply a phase" for Beatrice. They asserted that, given her previous autism spectrum diagnosis (new information for me), that it was common for her to have feelings of GD; however, this did not indicate an actual desire to transition. They refused to support Beatrice's desire to begin hormones and it was clear that without their support Beatrice would not be able to afford or manage a medical transition.

For Beatrice to begin hormone treatment under a physician's supervision, she needed a letter of support. Her physician had specifically asked that that I address the long-standing self-injury and substance abuse concerns that have been a constant part of Beatrice's life. Substance abuse and self-injury are both common clinical concerns in the trans community.[58,59] The presence of these concerns cannot be assumed to be a contraindication to treatment without further exploration and assessment on the part of the mental health provider. There are few, if any, empirically supported treatments to address these clinical concerns that are validated with gender diverse clients.

In this case, I wanted to provide support for this client; however, I had concerns about whether Beatrice would be able to manage her basic self-care. I consulted with other providers about this case and they shared my concerns about Beatrice's inability to manage her daily affairs. I did not write a letter to refer her to Dr Mason for initiation of hormone treatment. I spoke at length with Beatrice about my feelings that she was not ready to begin to hormones. This was a difficult conversation and she seemed to understand what was required for my reluctance to be resolved (eg, self-care). Although Beatrice stated that she understood this, her actions never changed. My work with Beatrice ended with a referral to another provider, in part

Due to my health needs. In this case, it was imperative that Beatrice have access to care; however, I needed to focus on my health needs.

## CLINICAL RECOMMENDATIONS

This article outlines 3 different clinical scenarios that highlight challenging situations. The following recommendations are offered to assist practitioners in their clinical decision-making regarding TGD clients:

- All mental health and medical providers should discuss the psychological impact of providing a diagnosis of GD or gender identity disorder to TGD clients. The authors recommend that all clinicians should have an open and honest conversation with clients regarding TGD-related diagnoses. This will assist with the therapeutic alliance and with an understanding of distress that may arise from the provision of the diagnosis.[20] Practitioners who diagnose their clients with GD or GID need to be prepared to discuss their viewpoints while validating any distress that the client may experience from the label. Hayne[60] recommends asking the following questions: "What is going on inside you right now because of hearing your diagnosis?" and "How has hearing your diagnosis affected you?" He posits that in cases in which clients are reticent to engage in ongoing discussion, it is important that clinicians continue to invite further dialogue and reassurance around this issue. If not, Hayne[60] suggests that clients often feel "passed over, evaded, and dismissed." The authors also recommend providing an explanation for why the diagnosis is required and to hear the fears the client may have based on receiving the diagnosis. It is likely that the provider can allay many of the fears the client may have.
- Clinicians are not required give a GD diagnosis unless someone requires the diagnosis in a letter. Many diagnostic labels remain controversial in the DSM-5.[51] There are no ethical codes that require a clinician to provide a diagnosis if the diagnosis does not fit the client's presenting concerns. The authors recommend that clinicians do not provide a diagnosis unless the diagnosis will provide medically necessary treatments for TGD clients.
- Clinicians and trainees will benefit from specific training in working with TDG clients. Graduate and other training programs should provide formal coursework for students to learn specific competencies in working with TGD individuals. Training should also be provided in how to consult with interdisciplinary health care providers. Many of the challenges that may exist for TGD clients could be reduced if their care providers were talking to each other about their care. As noted in the second case example, most trainees do not receive training on how to work effectively in team care.[54] It is likely that clinicians experience discomfort when needing to correct a microaggression or incorrect information about TGD identities and health care because research shows that diversity-related conversations rarely occur on health care teams.[61] The authors recommend that health care teams engage in TGD-related trainings together to ensure that the team members are on the same page with TGD health care which will prevent a member of the team from being the primary educator.
- Clinicians should always consult when a client is asking for a letter but may have co-occurring disorders that will delay or prevent the letter writing process. Consultation is a critical element to providing competent care. This is especially important for people who work in private practice and do not have the opportunity to engage in regular clinical staffing conversations. Too often, providers assume that once they are independently licensed that there is no need for ongoing

supervision or consultation. Although supervision, in the traditional sense, is no longer a required activity, consultation can, and should, be a part of a clinician's regular practice.

## REFERENCES

1. Coleman E, Bockting W, Botzer M, et al. Standards of care for the health of transsexual, transgender, and gender-nonconforming people, version 7. Int J Transgend 2012;13(4):166–232.
2. Colebunders B, De Cuypere G, Monstrey S. New criteria for sex reassignment surgery: WPATH standards of care, version 7, Revisited. Int J Transgend 2015; 16(4):222–33.
3. Dewey JM. Challenges of implementing collaborative models of decision making with trans-identified patients. Health Expect 2015;18(5):1508–18.
4. Radix A, Enisfeld J. Informed consent in transgender care. Perspectives from a US-based community health center. Z Sex Forsch 2014;27(1):31–43.
5. American Counseling Association. competencies for counseling with transgender clients. J LGBT Issues Couns 2010;4(3/4):135–59.
6. Singh AA, Burnes TR. Shifting the counselor role from gatekeeping to advocacy: ten strategies for using the competencies for counseling with transgender clients for individual and social change. J LGBT Issues Couns 2010;4(3–4):241–55.
7. Whitehead JC, Thomas J, Forkner B, et al. Reluctant gatekeepers: 'trans-positive' practitioners and the social construction of sex and gender. J Gend Stud 2012; 21(4):387–400.
8. Lev AI. Transgender emergence: therapeutic guidelines for working with gender-variant people and their families. New York: Routledge; 2013.
9. Levitt HM, Ippolito MR. Being transgender navigating minority stressors and developing authentic self-presentation. Psychol Women Q 2014;38(1):46–64.
10. Weber S. "Womanhood does not reside in documentation": queer and feminist student activism for transgender women's inclusion at women's colleges. J Lesbian Stud 2016;20(1):29–45.
11. Deutsch MB. Use of the informed consent model in the provision of cross-sex hormone therapy: a survey of the practices of selected clinics. Int J Transgend 2012; 13(3):140–6.
12. Stroumsa D. The state of transgender health care: policy, law, and medical frameworks. Am J Public Health 2014;104(3):e31–8.
13. Waltish S, Vance D, Fabricatore AN. Psychological evaluation of bariatric surgery applicants: procedures and reasons for delay or denial of surgery. Obes Surg 2007;17(12):1578–83.
14. Meyer W, Bockting WO, Cohen-Kettenis P, et al. The Harry Benjamin International Gender Dysphoria Association's standards of care for gender identity disorders, 6th version; 2001. Available at: http://www.cpath.ca/wp-content/uploads/2009/12/WPATHsocv6.pdf. Accessed October 31, 2016.
15. De Cuypere G, Vercruysse H Jr. Eligibility and readiness criteria for sex reassignment surgery: Recommendations for revision of the WPATH standards of care. Int J Transgend 2009;11(3):194–205.
16. Fraser L. Psychotherapy in the world professional association for Transgender Health's standards of care: background and recommendations. Int J Transgend 2009;11(2):110–26.
17. Lev AI. Gender dysphoria: two steps forward, one step back. Clin Soc Work J 2013;41(3):288–96.

18. Ellner D. Surgical treatments for the transgender population. In: Eckstrand K, Ehrenfeld JM, editors. Lesbian, gay, bisexual, and transgender healthcare. Switzerland: Springer International Publishing; 2016. p. 363–75.

19. Denson KE. Seeking support: transgender client experiences with mental health services. J Fem Fam Ther 2013;25(1):17–40.

20. Roller CG, Sedlak C, Draucker CB. Navigating the system: how transgender Individuals engage in health care services. J Nurs Scholarsh 2015;47(5):417–24.

21. Budge SL. Psychotherapists as gatekeepers: an evidence-based case study highlighting the role and process of letter writing for transgender clients. Psychotherapy (Chic) 2015;52(3):287–97.

22. Andresen EM, Malmgren JA, Carter WB, et al. Screening for depression in well older adults: evaluation of a short form of the CES-D (Center for Epidemiologic Studies Depression Scale). Am J Prev Med 1994;10:77–84.

23. Blais MA, Lenderking WR, Baer L, et al. Development and initial validation of a brief mental health outcome measure. J Pers Assess 1999;73:359–73.

24. Kessler RC, Berglund P, Demler O, et al. The epidemiology of major depressive disorder: results from the National Comorbidity Survey Replication (NCS-R). JAMA 2003;289:3095–105.

25. Watson JC, Schein J, McMullen E. An examination of clients' in-session changes and their relationship to the working alliance and outcome. Psychother Res 2010; 20(2):224–33.

26. Coolhart D, Baker A, Farmer S, et al. Therapy with transsexual youth and their families: a clinical tool for assessing youth's readiness for gender transition. J Marital Fam Ther 2013;39(2):223–43.

27. Coolhart D, Provancher N, Hager A, et al. Recommending transsexual clients for gender transition: a therapeutic tool for assessing readiness. J GLBT Fam Stud 2008;4(3):301–24.

28. Griffin L. The other dual role: therapist as advocate with transgender clients. J Gay Lesbian Ment Health 2011;15(2):235–6.

29. Holmes J, Freeman SB. Assessment and management of female-to-male transgender patients: a psychosocial and hormonal approach. Am J Nurse Pract 2012;16:6–14.

30. Pinto N, Moleiro C. Gender trajectories: transsexual people coming to terms with their gender identities. Prof Psychol Res Pr 2015;46(1):12.

31. Tishelman AC, Kaufman R, Edwards-Leeper L, et al. Serving transgender youth: challenges, dilemmas, and clinical examples. Prof Psychol Res Pr 2015;46(1): 307.

32. American Psychological Association. Guidelines for psychological practice with transgender and gender nonconforming people. Am Psychol 2015;70(9):832–64.

33. Irwig MS. Transgender care by endocrinologists in the United States. Endocr Pract 2016;22:832–6.

34. Ellis SJ, Bailey L, McNeil J. Trans people's experiences of mental health and gender identity services: a UK study. J Gay Lesbian Ment Health 2015;19(1): 4–20.

35. Riggs DW, Coleman K, Due C. Healthcare experiences of gender diverse Australians: a mixed-methods, self-report survey. BMC Public Health 2014;14:230.

36. Speer SA, McPhillips R. Patients' perspectives on psychiatric consultations in the Gender Identity Clinic: implications for patient-centered communication. Patient Educ Couns 2013;91(3):385–91.

37. Erich SA, Boutté-Queen N, Donnelly S, et al. Social work education: implications for working with the transgender community. Journal of Baccalaureate Social Work 2007;12(2):42–52.

38. Ali N, Fleisher W, Erickson J. Psychiatrists' and Psychiatry Residents' Attitudes Toward Transgender People. Acad Psychiatry 2016;40:268–73.

39. Bowers S, Lewandowski J, Savage TA, et al. School psychologists' attitudes toward transgender students. J LGBT Youth 2015;12(1):1–8.

40. Nisley E. Counseling professionals' attitudes toward transgender people and responses to transgender clients. Michigan: ProQuest Information & Learning; 2011.

41. Norton AT, Herek GM. Heterosexuals' attitudes toward transgender people: findings from a national probability sample of US adults. Sex roles 2013;68(11–12): 738–53.

42. Miller D, Spengler E, Spengler P. A meta-analysis of confidence and judgment accuracy in clinical decision making. J Couns Psychol 2015;62(4):553–67.

43. dickey lm, Budge SL, Katz-Wise SL, et al. Health disparities in the transgender community: exploring differences in insurance coverage. Psychol Sex Orientat Gend Divers. [advance online publication].

44. Poteat T, German D, Kerrigan D. Managing uncertainty: a grounded theory of stigma in transgender health care encounters. Soc Sci Med 2013;84:22–9.

45. Cruz TM. Assessing access to care for transgender and gender nonconforming people: a consideration of diversity in combating discrimination. Soc Sci Med 2014;110:65–73.

46. Ault A, Brzuzy S. Removing gender identity disorder from the Diagnostic and Statistical Manual of Mental Disorders: a call for action. Social Work 2009;54(2): 187–9.

47. Drescher J. Queer diagnoses: parallels and contrasts in the history of homosexuality, gender variance, and the Diagnostic and Statistical Manual. Arch Sex Behav 2010;39(2):427–60.

48. Langer SJ, Martin JI. How dresses can make you mentally ill: examining gender identity disorder in children. Child Adolesc Social Work J 2004;21(1):5–23.

49. Lev AI. The ten tasks of the mental health provider: recommendations for revision of the World Professional Association for Transgender Health's Standards of Care. Int J Transgend 2009;11(2):74–99.

50. Sennott SL. Gender disorder as gender oppression: a transfeminist approach to rethinking the pathologization of gender non-conformity. Women Ther 2010; 34(1–2):93–113.

51. American Psychiatric Association. APA DSM-5. DSM. 2013.

52. American Psychiatric Association. APA DSM-IV-TR. DSM. 2000.

53. Zucker K. The DSM-5 diagnostic criteria for gender dysphoria. In management of gender dysphoria. Springer Milan; 2015. p. 33–7.

54. Rosenman ED, Chandre JN, Ilgen JO, et al. Leadership training in health care action teams: a systematic review. Acad Med 2014;89(9):1295–306.

55. Schmaling KB, Giardino ND, Korslund KE, et al. The utility of interdisciplinary training and service: psychology training on a psychiatry consultation-liaison service. Prof Psychol Res Pr 2002;33(4):413.

56. Gómez-Gil E, Trilla A, Salamero M, et al. Sociodemographic, clinical, and psychiatric characteristics of transsexuals from Spain. Arch Sex Behav 2009;38(3): 378–92.

57. Murad MH, Elamin MB, Garcia MZ, et al. Hormonal therapy and sex reassign-ment: a systematic review and meta-analysis of quality of life and psychosocial outcomes. Clin Endocrinol 2010;72(2):214–31.
58. Cochran BN, Cauce AM. Characteristics of lesbian, gay, bisexual, and trans-gender individuals entering substance abuse treatment. J Subst Abuse Treat 2006;30(2):135–46.
59. dickey lm, Reisner SL, Juntunen CL. Non-suicidal self-injury in a large online sam-ple of transgender adults. Prof Psychol Res Pr 2015;46(1):3.
60. Hayne YM. Experiencing psychiatric diagnosis: client perspectives on being named mentally ill. J Psychiatr Ment Health Nurs 2003;10(6):722–9.
61. Dreachslin JL, Hunt PL, Sprainer E. Workforce diversity: implications for the effec-tiveness of health care delivery teams. Soc Sci Med 2000;50(10):1403–14.

# Hormonal and Surgical Treatment Options for Transgender Men (Female-to-Male)

 CrossMark

Ryan Nicholas Gorton, MD[a,b,]*, Laura Erickson-Schroth, MD, MA[c,d]

## KEYWORDS

- Transgender • Hormone replacement • Sex reassignment surgery
- Gender affirmation

## KEY POINTS

- Hormone therapy provides significant benefits, allowing many patients to live as male in society by 2 years of treatment.
- No increased risks of malignancy or cardiovascular end points with hormonal therapy are demonstrated in the literature, though minor increases might not be detectable at the current level of evidence.
- Mastectomy is the most common surgery necessary for transgender men as it significantly diminishes gender dysphoria, improves quality of life, and carries less risk than genital surgery.
- Individualized shared clinical decision-making is necessary, and clinicians should be able to provide the information needed for this process as provided by this review.

## INTRODUCTION

Hormone replacement therapy (HRT) and surgery for transgender people have existed for almost a century. However, of the more than 5200 citations in Medline referencing transgender care, fewer than 1000 were published before 1990. Transgender health remains a relatively young field, and the quality and quantity of evidence is limited. Guidelines such as those published by the World Professional Association for Transgender Health[1] (known as the WPATH Standards of Care) and the Endocrine Society[2]

Financial Disclosures: Neither author has a conflict of interest nor are they receiving any funding for this work.
[a] Lyon-Martin Health Services, 1748 Market Street, #201, San Francisco, CA 94102, USA; [b] Touro University California, 1310 Club Drive, Mare Island, Vallejo, CA 94592, USA; [c] Comprehensive Psychiatric Emergency Program, Mount Sinai Beth Israel, 10 Nathan D Perlman Place, New York, NY 10003, USA; [d] Hetrick-Martin Institute, 2 Astor Place, New York, NY 10003, USA
* Corresponding author.
E-mail address: nickgorton@gmail.com

Psychiatr Clin N Am 40 (2017) 79–97
http://dx.doi.org/10.1016/j.psc.2016.10.005
0193-953X/17/© 2016 Elsevier Inc. All rights reserved.

provide recommendations for care, though both recognize that the data are suboptimal and, thus, state that these are flexible recommendations especially when used by experienced clinicians. Care must be individualized, and not all patients need all treatments. For example, in a Dutch sample, only 58% of transgender men (transmen) who had decided on what treatment they would undertake requested full treatment (HRT, mastectomy, hysterectomy, and genital sex reassignment surgery [SRS]). Interestingly, the only universal request among patients was mastectomy, though only 2% declined testosterone (T). Reasons cited for not being interested in certain interventions were mostly related to surgical risks/outcomes but also included lack of genital dysphoria or a nonbinary gender identity.[3] Provider advocacy is also crucial for many patients to change identity documents and access sex-segregated facilities safely. Guidance for critically important letters can be found through the National Center for Transgender Equality (http://www.transequality.org/documents) and the Transgender Law Center (http://transgenderlawcenter.org/issues/id/id-please).

## Hormone Regimens

In the United States, HRT in transmen is typically T by intramuscular injection (IM) or transdermally. Subcutaneous (SQ) pellets are also an option, and in other countries oral formulations are available. Most commonly, T cypionate (Tc) (depot T) or enanthate (Te) are used parenterally. Recommended dosages are 200 to 400 mg per month, divided weekly to every other week.[2,4] Earlier onset (by 3 months of treatment) of desired effects may be greater in patients receiving higher doses, but these differences disappear at 12 months.[5]

IM Tc and Te can produce supraphysiologic levels of T 2 to 3 days after injection and subtherapeutic levels at trough (especially if given every other week rather than weekly). Transdermal T patches or gel, with dosages from 2.5 to 10 mg daily, may better mimic physiologic levels of T.[2,4] T can be transmitted to others by skin-to-skin contact; however, the amount transferred is modest.[6] The authors recommend patients not shower for at least 4 hours after application because it can significantly decrease serum T levels.[7] The authors also strongly caution patients around those most sensitive to transferred T (pregnant women and small children) to choose another method or be assiduous about keeping sites clothed for 4 hours after application.

Some transmen and providers use Tc or Te SQ, dosed weekly. There is scant research about this practice, with only 3 published articles[8–10] and 2 conference abstracts.[11,12] Although only 2 of these studies were in transmen, one was in youths aged 12 to 24 years, and all were limited by small sample size (137 patients total across all 5 studies), findings suggest that there is no difference in bioavailability between SQ and IM T. One study of SQ T noted that in obese patients serum T levels were more than 40% lower after 30 days than in nonobese patients, but this difference diminished at 4 months.[12] In patients for whom IM administration would carry other risks (for example, patients on warfarin) benefits of SQ dosing may outweigh the risks.

In addition to injected or transdermal T, adjuvant HRT treatments can be used. These treatments include progestagens, 5-α-reductase inhibitors (5-ARIs), aromatase inhibitors (AIs), gonadotropin-releasing hormone antagonists (GnRHas), and clitoral application of T. As shown in **Fig. 1**, administered T can be converted to dihydrotestosterone (DHT) by 5-α-reductase and to estrogens by aromatase. Higher DHT levels contribute to androgenic alopecia (AA) (ie, male pattern baldness) and increased estrogen to fat redistribution and other effects. The 5-ARIs are sometimes used by transmen to prevent further AA while on T. The authors do not usually recommend AIs despite the fact that T use only decreases serum E levels modestly. In most patients, there is no significant benefit to justify their risks, although they may be helpful in rare

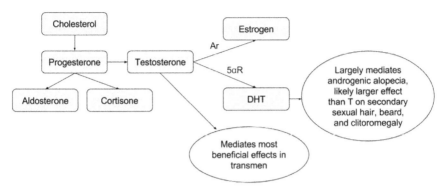

**Fig. 1.** Sex steroid metabolism. 5αR, 5-alpha reductase; Ar, aromatase; DHT, dihydrotestos-terone (cannot be aromatized into estrogen).

situations (eg, BrCa mutation carriers). Generally, GnRHas are too expensive for common use in adults.

*Treatment effects*
HRT mimics male puberty and can take 4 to 5 years to have full effect.[13] Although some effects like acne are purely negative, many are beneficial in some patients but undesired in others. For example, androgenic alopecia in a transman who otherwise has difficulty passing (being perceived by others as a cisgender man) might improve his passing and, thus, be welcome. Therefore, rather than subdivide effects into beneficial and harmful, the authors take a systems approach.

## SEXUAL AND REPRODUCTIVE EFFECTS AND MALIGNANCIES
### Physical Changes

Cessation of menses generally happens after 3 to 6 months on T[2,13–15] but is dose dependent. With lower doses, amenorrhea may take longer or not happen at all without the addition of progestagens, a GnRH agonist,[13] or endometrial ablation.[2] A progesterone-eluting intrauterine device (IUD) is an option for transmen who desire amenorrhea as well as contraception.

Clitoral growth may start as early as 3 months but generally peaks by 1 to 2 years at an average of 4.6 cm.[2,14] Clitoral length is important for some transmen, especially those who desire SRS. Given that topical DHT has modestly increased penile size in boys with congenital micropenis,[16] and the clitoris and penis are developmentally homologous, some patients and surgeons use topical DHT to enhance clitoromegaly. This practice is unstudied, and DHT is unavailable in the United States. Transmen may try topical T compounded into creams, but the amount used must be subtracted from other prescribed T to avoid supraphysiologic levels. Although also unstudied, some transmen and surgeons use suction devices to enhance growth. Patients choosing this should be cautioned to stop if it causes any pain. A study in Iran using a traction device after metoidioplasty reported longer length than previous studies, but attribution to the device is uncertain.[17]

### Sexuality

Transmen's sexuality requires significantly more investigation. One fairly well-documented phenomenon is the increase in libido that often, but not always, comes with initiating T and can be welcome or bothersome. A prospective study of 50

Transmen starting HRT showed that frequency of desire, masturbation, sexual fantasies, and arousal significantly increased after 1 year of HRT.[18] In a study of 45 transmen on HRT who had all undergone some type of gender-affirming surgery, 73.9% of the participants reported an increase in sexual desire after these interventions. Although no direct associations were found between T and sexual desire, those with elevated levels of luteinizing hormone (LH), indicating suboptimal T therapy, reported significantly lower solitary sexual desire levels. Suppressed LH, indicating sufficient T therapy, was associated with having greater need for sexual activities and more frequent excessive sexual desire.[19] Increased libido in transmen seems more significant when beginning T. In a cross-sectional study of 138 transmen, shorter duration of treatment was associated with higher sexual desire.[20]

The effect genital surgery may have on libido in transmen is less well understood. In the same cross-sectional study,[20] having undergone phalloplasty and/or implantation of an erection prosthesis did not affect sexual desire scores. Also of interest to many transmen regarding genital surgeries is the preservation of orgasmic potential. A 2009 review of research on sexual functioning after genital surgery indicates that ability to orgasm is likely preserved after genital surgery in transmen.[21] Specific genital surgeries are discussed later.

Transmen starting T sometimes report difficulties with pain during vaginal penetration, clitoral stimulation, or orgasm. Vaginal atrophy occurs, with diminished estrogen receptors in the vagina, as in menopausal women, making vaginal penetration more difficult for some. This atrophy may be noted as early as 3 months on T but may take 2 years to peak in effect.[2,22] For those who report pain after orgasm, the authors advise ibuprofen 1 hour before sexual activity.

Sexual orientation in transmen, and the effect of HRT, is a subject of increasing research. Baseline demographics regarding sexual orientation vary significantly depending on the population. In a 2013 study in Ontario, Canada, 63.3% of 227 transmen identified as gay or bisexual or reported having sex with other men.[23] Alternatively, a 2014 study conducted in Europe (Netherlands, Germany, Norway, Belgium) found that 80.4% of 172 transmen were attracted exclusively to women.[24]

Some transmen report their sexual orientation changes or broadens with social transition and/or starting T, though little data exist about this phenomenon. In a German study of 45 transmen, 73.4% reported initially being attracted to women exclusively. Twenty-two percent of all transmen reported a change in sexual orientation after HRT and/or surgery. Sixty percent of those whose orientation changed noted the change after starting T but before surgery. Those initially exclusively attracted to men were more likely to report a change in orientation after treatment.[25] In a community-based sample of 452 transgender and gender-nonconforming people in Massachusetts (not broken down by gender identity), among those who transitioned socially and/or medically/surgically, 64.6% reported a subsequent change in attractions. Transmasculine individuals were less likely than transfeminine individuals to report sexual fluidity.[26] There is still significant research needed in the area of sexual orientation and sexual orientation change in transmen.

### Reproduction

A 2012 survey of transmen in the Netherlands, all of whom had some type of transition-related surgery, showed transmen create families in a variety of different ways, and many desire to have children.[27] Transmen may have biological children before a hysterectomy or adopt, stepparent, have a child with a female partner and donated sperm, or any number of other ways of becoming a parent. Transmen interested in biological children should be aware of their options before making decisions about hormonal or surgical interventions.

There are conflicting results in the literature; however, most studies have shown increased rates of polycystic ovarian syndrome (PCOS) and/or hyperandrogenemia in transmen before starting HRT.[28–32] This finding suggests that transmen may have more difficulty conceiving even before T. Once started, T produces oligoovulation; but complete anovulation cannot be assumed. In a study of pregnancy in transmen, 20% conceived without resuming menstruation and 24% of pregnancies were unplanned.[33] Therefore, patients must understand that *T is not effective birth control*. For those who engage in penile-vaginal intercourse, contraception must be ensured, as T is a known teratogen and a Food and Drug Administration pregnancy category X drug (absolutely contraindicated in pregnancy). Should a transman become pregnant on HRT and wish to keep the pregnancy, T must be discontinued immediately and he should be referred to an obstetrician comfortable with both transgender clients and high-risk pregnancies. Progesterone-only birth control methods, such as implants, depot injections, and progesterone-releasing IUDs, are effective contraceptive methods for transmen.[34]

There is no doubt that some transmen with a history of T use have become pregnant (or donated ovum for their female partner's pregnancy) resulting in healthy babies, although there are little data about whether timing or duration of T use affects fertility. There are, however, no guarantees that fertility will be preserved. In a survey of 41 transmen who successfully delivered babies, 61% had used T at some point before conception. Among those who had taken T, 80% reported menstruation within 6 months of stopping. Twenty percent conceived while still amenorrheic from HRT. Ninety-six percent were pregnant within 6 months of stopping T. Pregnancy, delivery, and neonatal outcomes did not differ between those who had taken T before pregnancy and those who had not.[33] Because the sample size was small, further research is needed to understand whether there are differences in outcomes among larger populations.

Like T, genital surgeries can affect fertility, depending on the type of procedure. A hysterectomy and bilateral oophorectomy leads to irreversible sterility. Simple metoidioplasty without removal or closure of the vagina does not cause sterility, but postoperative changes could potentially make delivery more challenging.

Fertility preservation options for transmen include embryo, oocyte, and ovarian cryopreservation. The most reliable is embryo cryopreservation. This option requires ovarian stimulation with feminizing hormones, frequent vaginal US for monitoring, and transvaginal oocyte aspiration, which may be difficult for some transmen. A sperm donor must be chosen to proceed with embryo cryopreservation. Once preserved, embryos may be implanted in patients, a partner, or surrogate. Oocyte cryopreservation has the advantage that the sperm donor need not be chosen initially. However, it involves the same potentially uncomfortable procedures (feminizing hormones, vaginal US, and transvaginal aspiration) and is less reliable at producing viable pregnancies later. Ovarian tissue cryopreservation is currently experimental. It involves resection and freezing of ovarian tissue for later use. This procedure can be performed while on T and as a part of an already planned hysterectomy. Ovarian tissue transplants have resulted in viable pregnancies, but in vitro maturation of follicles is not yet possible.[34,35]

## Cancer Risk

Patients often express concern about gynecologic and breast cancers with HRT. Although some information is known about the risk, the authors simply do not have enough information to provide definitive answers to many questions about differential risk. No definite link between malignancy and T in transmen has been demonstrated.[36] Patients deserve the best information we have to make informed decisions even when the answer is that we do not know.

In animal models and in vitro studies, androgens inhibit breast cancer proliferation; women with hyperandrogenemia have no increase in breast cancer attributable to T.[37–39] Moreover, the largest follow-up study of transmen, encompassing 795 transgender men followed for a total of 15,974 person years (ie, total number of years that all participants have been in the study), demonstrated a breast cancer rate similar to male breast cancer risk, likely because most patients underwent mastectomy and the population was young.[40] Of the 16 reported cases in the literature of breast cancer in transmen, only 11 had taken T before the diagnosis, suggesting no evidence for a role of T. Mastectomy does not necessarily eliminate the risk, as not all breast tissue is removed. Of the 16 cases, 4 occurred after mastectomy, 2 were found at mastectomy, and 5 were in transmen unable to obtain mastectomy.[40–44]

A meta-analysis of risk in women with endogenous hyperandrogenemia (PCOS) showed an increase in the overall risk of endometrial cancer.[37] However, only 2 cases of endometrial cancer (one was an incidental carcinoma in situ) in transmen have been reported.[45,46] Two histopathologic studies of transmen after hysterectomy conflicted in that one showed half atrophic and half proliferative endometrium, whereas the other showed only atrophy.[45,47] Fortunately, endometrial cancer usually presents as postmenopausal vaginal bleeding. If amenorrheic transmen resume vaginal bleeding while on HRT, evaluation by ultrasonography, endometrial biopsy, or gynecologic consultation is necessary after more common causes are eliminated (eg, cervicitis, pregnancy, and low T levels).

To date, 3 cases of ovarian cancer in transmen have been reported in medical literature[48,49] and one transman with ovarian cancer was presented in the 2001 documentary *Southern Comfort*,[50] totaling 4 known cases. A systematic review and meta-analysis of malignancy risk in women with endogenous hyperandrogenemia (PCOS) showed no increase in overall risk of ovarian cancer.[37] Unfortunately, the true incidence in transmen is at present mathematically impossible to know.

Hormonal influences on cervical cancer are not well known. However, high-risk human papillomavirus (hrHPV) infection and inadequate screening dwarf the risk of hormonal influence. Rates of human papillomavirus may be increased because transmen do have higher rates of smoking.[15,51,52] The American College of Obstetricians and Gynecologists (ACOG) recommends that cervical cancer screening for transmen who retain a cervix should be the same age-appropriate screening as for cisgender women.[53] However, transmen are more likely to have inadequate cytology and take longer to follow up inadequate Papanicolaou tests than cisgender women even at a lesbian, gay, bisexual, and transgender (LGBT)–competent health center.[54] Some of this may be due to provider and patient discomfort; however, T causes vaginal atrophy; in the same study, duration on T was independently associated with inadequate cytology. After the Addressing the Need for Advanced HPV Diagnostics (ATHENA) study demonstrated hrHPV screening is more sensitive (although less specific) than cytology,[55] the ACOG's 2016 recommendations advise cytology every 3 years for women aged 21 to 29 years and cotesting every 5 years for women 30 to 65 years.[56] In transmen with difficult pelvic examinations, the authors recommend at a minimum cotesting in transmen of all ages; if hrHPV is negative, patients can be safely screened again in 3 years even if cytology returns inadequate. If either hrHPV or cytology is abnormal, standard algorithms should be followed.

## OTHER SYSTEMIC EFFECTS
### Hair and Skin

Acne is one of the earliest noticeable changes with T and peaks after 6 to 24 months.[2,57] Significant acne develops in 5% to 27% of transmen.[36,58–61] In addition to the face, acne of the back is common.[62] Although acne is mild or nonexistent in 94% of transmen after an average of 10 years on T,[57] scarring persists. For bothersome acne, the authors suggest standard treatments should be tried before decreasing the T dose if it is within the physiologic range.

In addition to HRT, as a result of tight breast binding, transmen may develop worse acne on the back and/or monilial dermatitis under breasts, especially in warm weather. Some patients are reticent to volunteer this fact, fearing the need to disrobe for an examination, so these complications should be inquired about, as treatments are simple and effective.

Noticeable facial and body hair usually occurs by the sixth month but may take up to 5 years to fully develop,[2,45] and considerable variation exists among transmen.[57,62] Needing to shave is present in 69% to 100% of patients by 2 years on T[58,60]; however, facial hair growth is unpredictable because of genetic variability.[14]

In addition to hair growth, AA may begin early in susceptible individuals but may occur at any time.[2] Given that patients generally start T at ages whereby AA is infrequent, only 5% report AA in the first year of treatment, though by 10 to 13 years 50% to 64% do.[57,63] Additionally, Wierckx[64] found that, although age correlated with AA, duration on T did not. Although treatments for AA, such as minoxidil and 5-ARIs, are effective in transmen, reduction of T dose may also diminish AA. A study of oophorectomized transmen on T alongside 5-ARIs showed lower DHT levels but also diminished lean muscle mass gain.[65] Transmen should also be counseled that secondary sexual hair development and clitoromegaly could be inhibited or delayed with use of 5-ARIs.

### Voice

T lengthens vocal cords and decreases fundamental frequency. Subtle changes may occur early. The voice may not stabilize until 1 to 3 years but generally reaches a normal male range.[2,13,66–68] As many as 1 in 4 transmen report vocal symptoms in the first 2 years, and these patients may benefit from speech therapy referral.[66]

### Musculoskeletal

Generally, muscle mass and strength increase and body fat decreases, but changes may not peak until the fifth year of T.[2,15,51,69,70] Unfortunately, visceral fat increases have been noted.[71] These parameters depend heavily on diet and physical activity, so healthy diet and exercise should be encouraged.

Transmen undergoing HRT before oophorectomy have modestly diminished serum E.[14,22,47,72–75] Studies of T and oophorectomy on bone mineral density (BMD) are mixed. With T, several studies show preserved BMD and increased markers of bone formation.[51,60,76] After oophorectomy, E levels are lower despite aromatization of some T to E. A study of oophorectomized transmen on T, as well as an AI, which further decreases E levels, demonstrated worsened BMD and markers of bone resorption.[65] Although some studies of transmen 5+ years after SRS on HRT showed no osteoporosis and preserved BMD,[77] Ruetsche and others[74,76,78] have demonstrated BMD may diminish despite HRT. Adding bisphosphonates may reverse this.[74] Higher LH levels after oophorectomy were inversely related to BMD, suggesting that adequate HRT could diminish the risk of osteoporosis.[76]

## Hematologic and Pulmonary

T increases hematocrit by increasing erythropoietin, and this is accentuated with IM T because of supraphysiologic peak levels.[13,77] This increase is usually small, and only 4% develop erythrocytosis using appropriately dosed T.[15,70]

One study showed significantly increased snoring among transmen after HRT and mastectomy despite decreased smoking rates from 46% to 30%.[18] Although new-onset sleep apnea should be in the differential for transmen with erythrocytosis, other studies demonstrated no sleep problems after 1 to 2 years of HRT.[15,60] In addition to the effects of T, tight breast binding may restrict pulmonary excursion.

### Vascular Disease and Risk Factors

The relationship between T and insulin resistance is not completely clear. Pre-HRT insulin resistance in transmen has been associated with obesity but not PCOS.[28] In 2 studies, T was linked to decreased insulin sensitivity but not increased fasting blood sugar or insulin.[71,80] Other studies showed no increase in insulin levels or insulin sensitivity on T.[15,19,72,75] Most studies demonstrate either no change or an increase in body mass index (BMI) in transmen after T,[71–73,75,81] with pre-HRT obesity as a risk factor for increased BMI after HRT.[58]

A meta-analysis of cardiovascular risk factors in transmen demonstrated worsening of triglycerides (TG) after HRT, a small but statistically significant decrease in high-density lipoprotein (HDL) cholesterol, and an increase in blood pressure, although the changes were so minor as to be of trivial clinical significance.[82] Subsequent studies demonstrated decreased HDL, increased TG, increased or unchanged total cholesterol and low-density lipoprotein cholesterol,[15,59,60,72,81,83] and no or trivial ($\leq$5 mm Hg) increases in systolic blood pressure.[15,59,60,81] In one of these studies, clinical hypertension developed in 6% of patients.[59]

Fortunately, no studies have demonstrated an increased risk of hard clinical end points of vascular disease in transmen.[36,84,85] Nonetheless, because of worsening surrogate markers and limitations of the research, reduction of other cardiovascular risks is advised.

## FOLLOW-UP AND SCREENING ON HORMONE REPLACEMENT THERAPY

The Endocrine Society's guidelines suggest clinical and laboratory monitoring every 3 months in the initial year of treatment, then every 6 to 12 months thereafter.[2] After the initial year, unless other health conditions indicate a need for closer follow-up, the authors find annual visits are adequate. In addition to the screening described earlier, providers should ask about smoking cessation and attempts, given the higher rates of smoking noted earlier. For LGBT smoking resources see https://smokefree. gov/lgbt-and-smoking. Providers with clinical questions about individual patients can consult the TransLine Clinical Consultation service: https://transline.zendesk. com/home. In addition, a summary table of hormone replacement therapy and monitoring for both transmen and transwomen is available at https://transline.zendesk. com/forums/23103088-Hormone-Therapy.

### Laboratory and Ancillary Testing

Laboratory test results should typically be interpreted with regard to normal male ranges for hematocrit, liver function tests (LFTs), and possibly creatinine.[15,75,76,86,87] Attribution of elevated LFTs to T should happen only after other causes are ruled out.

The Endocrine Society's guidelines recommend T be assessed midcycle and be between 350 and 700 ng/dL with injected T; levels can be taken at any time in transmen on topical T.[2] The Royal College of Psychiatrists London recommends testing at trough (before the next injection) and levels should be in or less than the lower range of normal for men.[88]

In truly low-resourced areas, with little if any laboratory testing available, the authors recommend that at a minimum after 6 months, blood sugar and hematocrit be checked and then rechecked every 2 years.

The Endocrine Society's guidelines suggest checking estradiol levels in transmen.[3] However, despite predictable decreases in estradiol, gonadotropins, and progesterone,[60,60] it is the authors' practice to do this only if a problem arises, such as unexplained vaginal bleeding or inadequate androgenization. With HRT, E diminishes only modestly.[14,22,47,72–75] In some transmen, awareness of residual E may exacerbate dysphoria despite adequate masculinization.

The authors agree with the Endocrine Society's guidelines that bone density should be monitored if risk factors exist, in patients after oophorectomy who cease HRT, and at 60 years of age.[2]

## SURGICAL TREATMENTS

There is no one-size-fits-all approach to surgery in transmen, and a minority of transmen choose not to undergo any type of surgery. For some patients, surgery is not covered by insurance and is out of reach financially. However, in those who do undergo surgery, it has been shown to improve mental health.[89–91] The Standards of Care published by WPATH provide guidance for referral of patients for surgery as well as referral for both surgery and medical treatment if the assessor is not also the prescribing provider. These standards are "intended to be flexible in order to meet the diverse health care needs of transsexual, transgender, and gender-nonconforming people."[1]

### Mastectomy and Hysterectomy

Many transmen even after sufficient HRT find it necessary to bind their breasts. Problems that result from binding include pain, diminished respiratory capacity, and skin irritation or infection.[92] Even with binding, many transmen require surgery in order to pass as male,[93] which is important to many but not all. Mastectomy has been shown to improve patients' ability to pass as male and their confidence in doing so.[94] The case for the medical necessity of mastectomy has been made elsewhere.[95] Mastectomy results in significantly diminished dysphoria even to the point that further surgeries may be unnecessary. In 2 studies, 38% to 45% of transmen who had undergone mastectomy declined or were undecided on whether to undergo genital SRS.[3,96]

Mastectomy technique depends on patient preference and a realistic assessment of breast size, ptosis (sagging), and skin elasticity. Periareolar mastectomy removes breast and adipose tissue through a partial or full incision around the areola. A limited amount of skin may be resected around the incision (in a doughnut shape). Periareolar mastectomy is appropriate for small, less ptotic breasts, with good elasticity. Inframammary (double incision [DI]) mastectomy is appropriate for larger breasts. DI includes procedures that keep the nipple on a dermal pedicle (to preserve protective and erotic sensation) or free nipple graft. DI often gives the best cosmetic result for transmen with larger breasts but leaves larger scars. In most who have free nipple grafts, protective sensation returns but may be incomplete. Complication rates for mastectomy are low (8%–25%), with most being minor and less than 10% requiring urgent reoperation (usually hematoma evacuations). From 3% to 32% of patients may need cosmetic revision, but satisfaction is high (79%–100%).[92,93,97–101]

Hysterectomy may be necessary for transmen to address their gender dysphoria, as a protective measure in those who are unwilling or unable to undergo routine gyneco logic screenings, or even for legal purposes, as some states/countries require this procedure to be allowed to change identity documents.[2] Hysterectomy/bilateral salpingo-oophorectomy (BSO) may be performed in conjunction with mastectomy without greater complications than have been reported in either alone.[100,102]

### Genital Surgery

Metoidioplasty and phalloplasty are the two primary options for transmen seeking genital surgery. Phalloplasty was originally developed in cisgender men suffering penile loss, whereas metoidioplasty was developed in transmen based on a variation of repair for severe hypospadias[103,104] Metoidioplasty moves the hypertrophied clitoris anteriorly to a normal penile position. Phalloplasty uses tissue from other parts of the body (donor site) to construct a neophallus as a pedicled or free flap. Both can include urethroplasty (extension of the urethra) and scrotoplasty with implantation of testicular prosthesis. Although numerous studies have shown poor quality-of-life (QOL) measures in transmen before treatment, studies of transmen undergoing genital SRS have shown global QOL scores indistinguishable from the general popula-tion.[90,91] To the authors' knowledge there are no studies demonstrating worsening QOL due to genital SRS.

Metoidioplasty is generally a single procedure and is lower cost than phalloplasty, with no need for a donor skin site.[94] It may or may not include urethral lengthening. Complications include spraying or dribbling in 28% (which often resolves spontane-ously) and urethral strictures or fistulas in 8% to 37%.[105–108] The ability to micturate while standing is reported in 30% to 100%. However, penetrative intercourse is rarely possible.[94] Erotic sensation, ability to orgasm, and erectile function is reported to be as high as 100%.[17,105] After 12 months on T, average stretched clitoral length increased from 1.4 to 4.6 cm[13] and reported average postoperative lengths range from 5.6 to 8.7 cm.[17,105] Patient satisfaction is high (83%–100%); however, some pa-tients go on to subsequent phalloplasty.[105,106,108]

Phalloplasty is a more difficult procedure with additional donor site morbidity. The radial forearm is considered the gold standard donor site because the radial artery provides excellent blood supply and the antebrachial cutaneous nerves can be anas tomosed to the ilioinguinal nerve for protective sensation and the dorsal clitoral nerves for erotic sensation.[94] The main disadvantage is donor site visibility and potential loss of sensation or function of the extremity. Other donor sites include the lower leg, abdomen, thigh, upper arm, scapula, and groin.[109–115] In patients after phalloplasty, ability to orgasm with masturbation and intercourse has been reported from 70% to 100%.[90,98,116–119] Patient satisfaction with phalloplasty ranges from 88% to 100%.[98,102,116,119–121] However, complication rates are significant, with urethral stric-ture or fistula formation in 11% to 80% (most studies are at or less than 40%), partial or complete graft necrosis in 0% to 18%, infection in 0% to 7%, and vascular thrombosis in 0% to 12%.[102,112,115,117,119–126] Many early fistulas resolve spontaneously, and the ability to micturate while standing is as high as 100%.[115,122,125] Fistulas are earlier complications; strictures generally occur later. The mean time between phalloplasty and stricture repair is almost 2 years, with a third of patients requiring more than one procedure.[127] Lifetime urologic follow-up is recommended.[94] Postvoid inconti-nence or dribbling occurs in half of those who undergo phalloplasty due to the virtual space of the neourethra filling with urine.[122] Patients can press up roughly on the lowest part of the urethra (usually at the scrotum), with 75% learning to expel residual urine.[128]

Scrotoplasty (creating a scrotum from the labia majora with testicular prostheses) is generally done with phalloplasty or metoidioplasty and causes fewer complications than the primary surgery. However, loss or displacement of prostheses occurs in 2% to 30% and can increase risk of urethral complications.[102,106,108,129,130]

## QUALITY OF LIFE AND PSYCHOLOGICAL WELL-BEING WITH HORMONE REPLACEMENT THERAPY AND/OR SURGICAL INTERVENTIONS

One of the most important goals of hormonal and surgical interventions in transmen is to treat gender dysphoria, and there is ample evidence that these are effective. A 2010 meta-analysis showed that 86% of transmen had significant improvement in gender dysphoria with hormonal treatment and 78% had significant improvement in QOL, although in 23 of the 28 studies reviewed, patients had undergone both SRS and HRT, making it somewhat difficult to separate the effects of T versus surgeries.[131] A subsequent systematic review of HRT on psychological functioning and QOL in transgender people found 3 additional prospective cohort studies published after this first analysis, which together included 67 transmen.[132] Two of the studies showed an improvement in psychological functioning (depression, anxiety, and global functioning) at 3 to 6 months and 12 months of treatment for both transmen and transwomen.[133,134] The third study found an improvement in QOL for both groups, but this was statistically significant for transwomen only.[135]

Regarding surgical treatments, a large, Internet-based survey of 446 transmen found that those who had undergone mastectomy reported higher QOL than those who had not.[89] Other studies compared transmen undergoing surgeries with control, nonclinical populations. Transmen have been shown to have high rates of mental health issues compared with the general population.[136] Therefore, comparisons to the general population that show transmen to be similar demonstrate that they have better-than-expected functioning. In a cross-sectional study of 49 transmen, 94% of whom had phalloplasties, an average of 8 years after surgeries, there were no differences in the rates of psychological problems compared with the reference Belgian population.[90] Similarly, in a study of 14 transmen, 11 of whom had phalloplasties, 2 years after surgery, there was no difference in QOL scores from a control group of cisgender men.[91]

Starting the transition process in young adulthood, when appropriate, has also been shown to be beneficial. A 2014 study in the Netherlands demonstrated that, for those patients treated in puberty, dysphoria resolved; on measures of psychological function, transgender young adults were indistinguishable from age-matched controls.[137]

The evidence, though limited, demonstrates both HRT and surgical interventions benefit mental health, decrease suicide, and improve QOL and that HRT is generally safe in transmen. Unfortunately, double blinding is impossible and a randomized controlled study is at this point unethical given the known benefits of treatment and the high risk of suicide in untreated patients. In addition, low regret rates (generally 0%–3%) and significantly diminished suicidality across several studies speak to the benefits gained with treatment.[138–140]

## SUMMARY

From a medical provider's point of view, hormonal treatment of transmen is relatively straightforward; no increase in hard clinical end points for serious complications like irreversible diseases or malignancy have been demonstrated. Surgery, although imperfect, provides significant relief of gender dysphoria. There remain many unanswered research questions, but provision of medical and surgical care to transmen provides lifelong benefits with regard to mental health symptoms and QOL; these treatments are both medically necessary and highly rewarding to both patients and providers. The first few years of transition can be a time of intense adjustment but allow patients to finally live lives whereby society accepts their sense of self and gender identity.

## REFERENCES

1. Coleman E, Bockting W, Botzer M, et al. Standards of care, for the health of transsexual, transgender, and gender nonconforming people. Int J Transgend 2012;13(4):165–232.
2. Hembree WC, Cohen-Kettenis P, Delemarre-Van De Waal HA, et al. Endocrine treatment of transsexual persons: an Endocrine Society clinical practice guideline. J Clin Endocrinol Metab 2009;94(9):3132–54.
3. Beek TF, Kreukels BPC, Cohen-Kettenis PT, et al. Partial treatment requests and underlying motives of applicants for gender affirming interventions. J Sex Med 2015;12(11):2201–5.
4. Meriggiola MC, Gava G. Endocrine care of transpeople part I. A review of cross? Sex hormonal treatments, outcomes and adverse effects in transmen. Clin Endocrinol (Oxf) 2015;83(5):597–606.
5. Nakamura A, Watanabe M, Sugimoto M, et al. Dose-response analysis of testosterone replacement therapy in patients with female to male gender identity disorder. Endocr J 2013;60(3):275–81.
6. De Ronde W. Hyperandrogenism after transfer of topical testosterone gel: case report and review of published and unpublished studies. Hum Reprod 2009; 24(2):425–8.
7. de Ronde W, Vogel S, Bui HN, et al. Reduction in 24-hour plasma testosterone levels in subjects who showered 15 or 30 minutes after application of testosterone gel. Pharmacotherapy 2011;31(3):248–52.
8. Al-Futaisi A, Al-Zakwani I. Subcutaneous administration of testosterone. Saudi Med J 2006;27(12):1843–6. Available at: http://ipac.kacst.edu.sa/eDoc/2006/161440_1.pdf.
9. Kaminetsky J, Jaffe JS, Swerdloff RS. Pharmacokinetic profile of subcutaneous testosterone enanthate delivered via a novel, prefilled single-use autoinjector: a phase II study. Sex Med 2015;3(4):269–79.
10. Olson J, Schrager SM, Clark LF, et al. Subcutaneous testosterone: an effective delivery mechanism for masculinizing young transgender men. LGBT Health 2014;1(3):165–7.
11. Boh B, Turco JH, Comi RJ. New and improved testosterone administration: a clinical case series of subcutaneous testosterone use in 26 transsexual males. Presented at the Endocrine Society's 97th Annual Meeting and Expo. San Diego, March 5–8, 2015.
12. Marotte J, Stout R, Alobuia W, et al. Use of a novel subcutaneous needle-free technique to deliver testosterone in hypogonadal men. J Sex Med 2015; 12(Suppl 1):12.
13. Seal LJ. A review of the physical and metabolic effects of cross-sex hormonal therapy in the treatment of gender dysphoria. Ann Clin Biochem 2016; 53(Pt 1):10–20.

14. Meyer WJ III, Finkelstein JW, Stuart CA, et al. Physical and hormonal evaluation of transexual patients during hormonal therapy. Arch Sex Behav 1986;15(2): 121–38.

15. Wierckx K, Van Caenegem E, Schreiner T, et al. Cross-sex hormone therapy in trans persons is safe and effective at short-time follow-up: results from the European network for the investigation of gender incongruence. J Sex Med 2014. http://dx.doi.org/10.1111/jsm.12571.

16. Choi SK, Han SW, Kim DH, et al. Transdermal dihydrotestosterone therapy and its effects on patients with microphallus. J Urol 1993;150(2):657–60.

17. Cohanzad S. Extensive metoidioplasty as a technique capable of creating a compatible analogue to a natural penis in female transsexuals. Aesthetic Plast Surg 2016;40(1):130–8.

18. Costantino A, Cerpolini S, Alvisi S, et al. A prospective study on sexual function and mood in female-to-male transsexuals during testosterone administration and after sex reassignment surgery. J Sex Marital Ther 2013;39(4):321–35.

19. Wierckx K, Elaut E, Van Caenegem E, et al. Sexual desire in female-to-male transsexual persons: exploration of the role of testosterone administration. Eur J Endocrinol 2011. http://dx.doi.org/10.1530/EJE-11-0250.

20. Wierckx K, Elaut E, Van Hoorde B, et al. Sexual desire in trans persons: associations with sex reassignment treatment. J Sex Med 2014;11(1):107–18.

21. Klein C, Gorzalka BB. Sexual functioning in transsexuals following hormone therapy and genital surgery: a review. J Sex Med 2009;6(11):2922–39.

22. Baldassarre M, Giannone FA, Foschini MP, et al. Effects of long-term high dose testosterone administration on vaginal epithelium structure and estrogen receptor-$\alpha$ and -$\beta$ expression of young women. Int J Impot Res 2013;25(5):172–7.

23. Bauer GR, Redman N, Bradley K, et al. Sexual health of trans men who are gay, bisexual, or who have sex with men: results from Ontario, Canada. Int J Transgend 2013;14(2):66–74.

24. Cerwenka S, Nieder TO, Cohen-Kettenis P, et al. Sexual behavior of gender-dysphoric individuals before gender-confirming interventions: a European multicenter study. J Sex Marital Ther 2014;40(5):457–71.

25. Auer MK, Fuss J, Höhne NN, et al. Transgender transitioning and change of self-reported sexual orientation. PLoS One 2014. http://dx.doi.org/10.1371/journal.pone.0110016.

26. Katz-Wise SL, Reisner SL, Hughto JW, et al. Differences in sexual orientation diversity and sexual fluidity in attractions among gender minority adults in Massachusetts. J Sex Res 2015;4499(July):1–11.

27. Wierckx K, Van Caenegem E, Pennings G, et al. Reproductive wish in transsexual men. Hum Reprod 2012;27(2):483–7.

28. Baba T, Endo T, Honnma H, et al. Association between polycystic ovary syndrome and female-to-male transsexuality. Hum Reprod 2007;22(4):1011–6.

29. Balen AH, Schachter ME, Montgomery D, et al. Polycystic ovaries are a common finding in untreated female to male transsexuals. Clin Endocrinol (Oxf) 1993; 38(3):325–9.

30. Becerra-Fernández A, Pérez-López G, Menacho Román M, et al. Prevalence of hyperandrogenism and polycystic ovary syndrome in female to male transsexuals. Endocrinol Nutr 2014;61(7):351–8.

31. Futterweit W, Weiss RA, Fagerstrom RM. Endocrine evaluation of forty female-to-male transsexuals: increased frequency of polycystic ovarian disease in female transsexualism. Arch Sex Behav 1986;15(1):69–78.

32. Bosinski HAG, Peter M, Bonatz G, et al. A higher rate of hyperandrogenic disorders in female-to-male transsexuals. Psychoneuroendocrinology 1997. http://dx.doi.org/10.1016/S0306-4530(97)00033-4.

33. Light AD, Obedin Malivor J, Sevelius JM, et al. Transgender men who experienced pregnancy after female-to-male gender transitioning. Obstet Gynecol 2014;124(6):1120–7.

34. De Roo C, Tilleman K, T'Sjoen G, et al. Fertility options in transgender people. Int Rev Psychiatry 2016;28(1):112–9.

35. Wallace SA, Blough KL, Kondapalli LA. Fertility preservation in the transgender patient expanding oncofertility care beyond cancer. Gynecol Endocrinol 2014; 30(12):868–71.

36. Bourgeois AL, Auriche P, Palmaro A, et al. Risk of hormonotherapy in transgender people: literature review and data from the French Database of Pharmacovigilance. Ann Endocrinol (Paris) 2016;77(1):14–21.

37. Barry JA, Azizia MM, Hardiman PJ. Risk of endometrial, ovarian and breast cancer in women with polycystic ovary syndrome: a systematic review and meta-analysis. Hum Reprod Update 2014;20(5):748–58.

38. Shufelt CL, Braunstein GD. Testosterone and the breast. Menopause Int 2008; 14(3):117–22.

39. Traish AM, Fetten K, Miner M, et al. Testosterone and risk of breast cancer: appraisal of existing evidence. Horm Mol Biol Clin Investig 2010;2(1):177–90.

40. Gooren LJ, van Trotsenburg MA, Giltay EJ, et al. Breast cancer development in transsexual subjects receiving cross-sex hormone treatment. J Sex Med 2013; 10:3129–34.

41. Brown GR. Breast cancer in transgender veterans a ten-case series. LGBT Health 2015;2(1):77–80.

42. Burcombe RJ, Makris A, Pittam M, et al. Breast cancer after bilateral subcutaneous mastectomy in a female-to-male trans-sexual. Breast 2003. http://dx.doi.org/10.1016/S0960-9776(03)00033-X.

43. Gooren L, Bowers M, Lips P, et al. Five new cases of breast cancer in transsexual persons. Andrologia 2015. http://dx.doi.org/10.1111/and.12399.

44. Nikolic DV, Djordjevic ML, Granic M, et al. Importance of revealing a rare case of breast cancer in a female to male transsexual after bilateral. World J Surg Oncol 2012;10:280.

45. Grynberg M, Fanchin R, Dubost G, et al. Histology of genital tract and breast tissue after long-term testosterone administration in a female-to-male transsexual population. Reprod Biomed Online 2010. http://dx.doi.org/10.1016/j.rbmo.2009.12.021.

46. Urban RR, Teng NNH, Kapp DS. Gynecologic malignancies in female-to-male transgender patients: the need of original gender surveillance. Am J Obstet Gynecol 2011. http://dx.doi.org/10.1016/j.ajog.2010.12.057.

47. Perrone AM, Cerpolini S, Maria Salfi NC, et al. Effect of long-term testosterone administration on the endometrium of female-to-male (FTM) transsexuals. J Sex Med 2009;6:3193–200.

48. Dizon DS, Tejada-Berges T, Koelliker S, et al. Ovarian cancer associated with testosterone supplementation in a female-to-male transsexual patient. Gynecol Obstet Invest 2006;62:226–8.

49. Hage JJ, Dekker JJML, Karim RB, et al. Ovarian cancer in female-to-male transsexuals: report of two cases. Gynecol Oncol 2000;76(3):413–5. Nick@lyon-martin.org.

50. Davis K. Southern comfort. HBO documentary. 2001.

51. Van Caenegem E, Wierckx K, Taes Y, et al. Body composition, bone turnover, and bone mass in trans men during testosterone treatment: 1-year follow-up data from a prospective case-controlled study (ENIGI). Eur J Endocrinol 2015. http://dx.doi.org/10.1530/EJE-14-0586.

52. Ott J, Kaufmann U, Bentz EK, et al. Incidence of thrombophilia and venous thrombosis in transsexuals under cross-sex hormone therapy. Fertil Steril 2010;93(4):1267–72.

53. Committee on Health Care for Underserved Women. Committee opinion No 512: health care for transgender individuals. Obstet Gynecol 2011;118(6): 1454–8.

54. Peitzmeier SM, Reisner SL, Harigopal P, et al. Female-to-male patients have high prevalence of unsatisfactory paps compared to non-transgender females: implications for cervical cancer screening. J Gen Intern Med 2014. http://dx.doi.org/10.1007/s11606-013-2753-1.

55. Wright TC, Stoler MH, Behrens CM, et al. Primary cervical cancer screening with human papillomavirus: end of study results from the ATHENA study using HPV as the first-line screening test. Gynecol Oncol 2015;136(2):189–97.

56. Practice bulletin: cervical cancer screening and prevention. Obstet Gynecol 2016 Dec;127(1):185–7.

57. Wierckx K, Van de Peer F, Verhaeghe E, et al. Short- and long-term clinical skin effects of testosterone treatment in trans men. J Sex Med 2014;11:222–9.

58. Asscheman H, Gooren LJG, Eklund PLE. Mortality and morbidity in transsexual patients with cross-gender hormone treatment. Metabolism 1989;38(9):869–73.

59. Mueller A, Kiesewetter F, Binder H, et al. Long-term administration of testosterone undecanoate every 3 months for testosterone supplementation in female-to-male transsexuals. J Clin Endocrinol Metab 2007;92(9):3470–5.

60. Mueller A, Haeberle L, Zollver H, et al. Effects of intramuscular testosterone undecanoate on body composition and bone mineral density in female-to-male transsexuals. J Sex Med 2010;7(9):3190–8.

61. van Kesteren PJ, Asscheman H, Megens JA, et al. Mortality and morbidity in transsexual subjects treated with cross-sex hormones. Clin Endocrinol (Oxf) 1997;47(3):337–42.

62. Giltay EJ, Gooren LJG. Effects of sex steroid deprivation/administration on hair growth and skin sebum production in transsexual. J Clin Endocrinol Metab 2014;85(8):2013–21.

63. Tangpricha V, Ducharme SH, Barber TW, et al. Endocrinologic treatment of gender identity disorders. Endocr Pract 2003;9(1):12–21.

64. Wierckx K, Van de Peer F, Verhaeghe E, et al. Short- and long-term clinical skin effects of testosterone treatment in trans men. J Sex Med 2014;11:222–9.

65. Meriggiola MC, Armillotta F, Costantino A, et al. Effects of testosterone undecanoate administered alone or in combination with letrozole or dutasteride in female to male transsexuals. J Sex Med 2008. http://dx.doi.org/10.1111/j.1743-6109.2008.00909.x.

66. Nygren U, Nordenskjöld A, Arver S, et al. Effects on voice fundamental frequency and satisfaction with voice in trans men during testosterone treatment—a longitudinal study. J Voice 2015. [Epub ahead of print].

67. Deuster D, Matulat P, Knief A, et al. Voice deepening under testosterone treatment in female-to-male gender dysphoric individuals. Eur Arch Otorhinolaryngol 2016;273(4):959–65.

68. Oregone M, Meli Di ... et al. Wide in [vocaleconionale transsexual persons after long-term androgen therapy. Laryngoscope 2014;124(6): 1409–14.

69. Haraldsen IR, Haug E, Falch J, et al. Cross-sex pattern of bone mineral density in early onset gender identity disorder. Horm Behav 2007. http://dx.doi.org/10.1016/j.yhbeh.2007.05.012.

70. Elbers JMH, de Jong S, Teerlink T, et al. Changes in fat cell size and in vitro lipolytic activity of abdominal and gluteal adipocytes after a one-year cross-sex hormone administration in transsexuals. Metabolism 1999;48(11):1371–7.

71. Elbers JMH, Giltay EJ, Teerlink T, et al. Effects of sex steroids on components of the insulin resistance syndrome in transsexual subjects. Clin Endocrinol (Oxf) 2003;58(5):562–71.

72. Cupisti S, Giltay EJ, Gooren LJ, et al. The impact of testosterone administration to female-to-male transsexuals on insulin resistance and lipid parameters compared with women with polycystic ovary syndrome. Fertil Steril 2010; 94(7):2647–53.

73. Deutsch MB, Bhakri V, Kubicek K. Effects of cross-sex hormone treatment on transgender women and men. Obstet Gynecol 2015;125(3):605–10.

74. Miyajima T, Kim YT, Oda H. A study of changes in bone metabolism in cases of gender identity disorder. J Bone Miner Metab 2012. http://dx.doi.org/10.1007/s00774-011-0342-0.

75. Giltay EJ, Hoogeveen EK, Elbers JM, et al. Effects of sex steroids on plasma total homocysteine levels: a study in transsexual males and females. J Clin Endocrinol Metab 1998;83(2):550–3.

76. Van Kesteren P, Lips P, Gooren LJG, et al. Long-term follow-up of bone mineral density and bone metabolism in transsexuals treated with cross-sex hormones. Clin Endocrinol (Oxf) 1998. http://dx.doi.org/10.1046/j.1365-2265.1998.00396.x.

77. Wierckx K, Mueller S, Weyers S, et al. Long-term evaluation of cross-sex hormone treatment in transsexual persons. J Sex Med 2012;9(10):2641–51.

78. Ruetsche AG, Kneubuehl R, Birkhaeuser MH, et al. Cortical and trabecular bone mineral density in transsexuals after long-term cross-sex hormonal treatment: a cross-sectional study. Osteoporos Int 2005;16(7):791–8.

79. Chandra P, Basra SS, Chen TC, et al. Alterations in lipids and adipocyte hormones in female-to-male transsexuals. Int J Endocrinol 2010;18:1–4.

80. Polderman KH, Gooren LJ, Asscheman H, et al. Induction of insulin resistance by androgens and estrogens. J Clin Endocrinol Metab 1994;79(1):265–71.

81. Quirós C, Patrascioiu I, Mora M, et al. Effect of cross-sex hormone treatment on cardiovascular risk factors in transsexual individuals. Experience in a specialized unit in Catalonia. Endocrinol Nutr 2015;62(5):210–6.

82. Elamin MB, Garcia MZ, Murad MH, et al. Effect of sex steroid use on cardiovascular risk in transsexual individuals: a systematic review and meta-analyses. Clin Endocrinol (Oxf) 2010. http://dx.doi.org/10.1111/j.1365-2265.2009.03632.x.

83. Ott J, Aust S, Promberger R, et al. Cross-sex hormone therapy alters the serum lipid profile: a retrospective cohort study in 169 transsexuals. J Sex Med 2011; 8(8):2361–9.

84. Gooren LJ. Management of female-to-male transgender persons: medical and surgical management, life expectancy. Curr Opin Endocrinol Diabetes Obes 2014;21(3):233–8.

85. Gooren LJ, Wierckx K, Giltay EJ. Cardiovascular disease in transsexual persons treated with cross-sex hormones: reversal of the traditional sex difference in cardiovascular disease pattern. Eur J Endocrinol 2014;170:809–19.

86. Van Caenegem E, Wierckx K, Taes Y, et al. Bone mass, bone geometry, and body composition in female-to-male transsexual persons after long-term cross-sex hormonal therapy. J Clin Endocrinol Metab 2012;97(7):2503–11.

87. Schlatterer K, Yassouridis A, von Werder K, et al. A follow-up study for estimating the effectiveness of a cross-gender hormone substitution therapy on transsexual patients. Arch Sex Behav 1998;27(5):475–92.

88. Royal College of Psychiatrists. Good practice guidelines for the assessment and treatment of adults with gender dysphoria. London: Royal College of Psychiatrists; 2013. Available at: http://www.rcpsych.ac.uk/usefulresources/publications/collegereports/cr/cr181.aspx. Accessed January 2, 2016.

89. Newfield E, Hart S, Dibble S, et al. Female-to-male transgender quality of life. Qual Life Res 2006;15(9):1447–57.

90. Wierckx K, Van Caenegem E, Elaut E, et al. Quality of life and sexual health after sex reassignment surgery in transsexual men. J Sex Med 2011;8(12):3379–88.

91. Castellano E, Crespi C, Dell'Aquila C, et al. Quality of life and hormones after sex reassignment surgery. J Endocrinol Invest 2015;38:1373–81.

92. Monstrey S, Selvaggi G, Ceulemans P, et al. Chest-wall contouring surgery in female-to-male transsexuals: a new algorithm. Plast Reconstr Surg 2008; 121(3):849–59.

93. Berry MG, Curtis R, Davies D. Female-to-male transgender chest reconstruction: a large consecutive, single-surgeon experience. J Plast Reconstr Aesthet Surg 2012;65:711–9.

94. Monstrey SJ, Ceulemans P, Hoebeke P. Sex reassignment surgery in the female-to-male transsexual. Semin Plast Surg 2011;25:229–44.

95. Richards C, Barrett J. The case for bilateral mastectomy and male chest contouring for the female-to-male transsexual. Ann R Coll Surg Engl 2013;95(2): 93–5.

96. Aydin D, Buk LJ, Partoft S, et al. Transgender surgery in Denmark from 1994 to 2015: 20-year follow-up study. J Sex Med 2016;13(4):720–5.

97. Bjerrome Ahlin H, Kolby L, Elander A. Improved results after implementation of the Ghent algorithm for subcutaneous mastectomy in female-to-male transsexuals. J Plast Surg Hand Surg 2014;48:362–7.

98. De Cuypere G, T'Sjoen G, Beerten R, et al. Sexual and physical health after sex reassignment surgery. Arch Sex Behav 2005. http://dx.doi.org/10.1007/s10508-005-7926-5.

99. Namba Y, Watanabe T, Kimata Y. Mastectomy in female-to-male transsexuals. Acta Med Okayama 2009;63(5):243–7.

100. Ott J, van Trotsenburg M, Kaufmann U, et al. Combined hysterectomy/salpingo-oophorectomy and mastectomy is a safe and valuable procedure for female-to-male transsexuals. J Sex Med 2010;7(6):2130–8.

101. Wolter A, Diedrichson J, Scholz T, et al. Sexual reassignment surgery in female-to-male transsexuals an algorithm for subcutaneous mastectomy. J Plast Reconstr Aesthet Surg 2015;68:184–91.

102. Schaff J. A new protocol for complete phalloplasty with free sensate and prelaminated osteofasciocutaneous flaps: experience in 37 patients. Microsurgery 2009;29:413–9.

103. Edgerton MT, Knorr NJ, Callison JR. The surgical treatment of transsexual patients: limitations and indications. Plast Reconstr Surg 1970;45(1):38–46.

104. Perovic SV, Djordjevic ML. Metoidioplasty: a variant of phalloplasty in female transsexuals. BJU Int 2003;92:981–5.

105. Djordjevic ML, Bizic MR. Comparison of two different methods for urethral lengthening in female to male (metoidioplasty) surgery. J Sex Med 2013; 10(5):1431–8.

106. Hage JJ, van Turnhout AA. Long-term outcome of metaidoioplasty in 70 female-to-male transsexuals. Ann Plast Surg 2006;57(3):312–6.

107. Takamatsu A, Harashina T. Labial ring flap: a new flap for metaidoioplasty in female-to-male transsexuals. J Plast Reconstr Aesthet Surg 2009;62(3):318–25.

108. Vukadinovic V, Stojanovic B, Majstorovic M, et al. The role of clitoral anatomy in female to male sex reassignment surgery. ScientificWorldJournal 2014;2014: 437378.

109. Dabernig J, Chan LKW, Schaff J. Phalloplasty with free (septocutaneous) fibular flap sine fibula. J Urol 2006;176:2085–8.

110. Hage JJ, Bloem JJAM, Suliman H. Review of the literature on techniques for phalloplasty with emphasis on the applicability in female-to-male transsexuals. J Urol 1993;150:1093–8.

111. Khouri RK, Young VL, Casoli VM. Long-term results of total penile reconstruction with a prefabricated lateral arm free flap. J Urol 1998;160:383–8.

112. Papadopulos NA, Schaff J, Biemer E. The use of free prelaminated and sensate osteofasciocutaneous fibular flap in phalloplasty. Injury 2008;39(3 suppl.):54–9.

113. Rubino C, Figus A, Dessy LA, et al. Innervated island pedicled anterolateral thigh flap for neo-phallic reconstruction in female-to-male transsexuals. J Plast Reconstr Aesthet Surg 2009;62:e45–9.

114. Terrier J-É, Courtois F, Ruffion A, et al. Surgical outcomes and patients' satisfaction with suprapubic phalloplasty. J Sex Med 2014;11(1):288–98.

115. Yang M, Zhao M, Li S, et al. Penile reconstruction by the free scapular flap and malleable penis prosthesis. Ann Plast Surg 2007;59(1):95–101.

116. Garcia MM, Christopher NA, De Luca F, et al. Overall satisfaction, sexual function, and the durability of neophallus dimensions following staged female to male genital gender confirming surgery: the Institute of Urology, London U.K. experience. Transl Androl Urol 2014;3(2):156–62.

117. Kim SK, Moon JB, Heo J, et al. A new method of urethroplasty for prevention of fistula in female-to-male gender reassignment surgery. Ann Plast Surg 2010; 64(6):759–64.

118. Selvaggi G, Monstrey S, Ceulemans P, et al. Genital sensitivity after sex reassignment surgery in transsexual patients. Ann Plast Surg 2007;58:427–33.

119. Song C, Wong M, Wong CH, et al. Modifications of the radial forearm flap phalloplasty for female-to-male gender reassignment. J Reconstr Microsurg 2011; 27(2):115–20.

120. Garaffa G, Christopher NA, Ralph DJ. Total phallic reconstruction in female-to-male transsexuals. Eur Urol 2010;57(4):715–22.

121. Kim SK, Lee KC, Kwon YS, et al. Phalloplasty using radial forearm osteocutaneous free flaps in female-to-male transsexuals. J Plast Reconstr Aesthet Surg 2009;62:309–17.

122. Hoebeke P, Selvaggi G, Ceulemans P, et al. Impact of sex reassignment surgery on lower urinary tract function. Eur Urol 2005;47(3):398–402.

123. Leriche A, Timsit MO, Morel-Journel N, et al. Long-term outcome of forearm flee-flap phalloplasty in the treatment of transsexualism. BJU Int 2008;101(10): 1297–300.

124. Monstrey S, Hoebeke P, Dhont M, et al. Surgical therapy in transsexual patients: a multi-disciplinary approach. Acta Chir Belg 2001;101:200–9.

125. Zhang Y-F, Liu CY, Qu CY, et al. Is vaginal mucosal graft the excellent substitute material for urethral reconstruction in female-to-male transsexuals? World J Urol 2015;33:2115–23.
126. Vriens JPM, Acosta R, Soutar DS, et al. Recovery of sensation in the radial forearm free flap in oral reconstruction. Plast Reconstr Surg 1996;98:649–56.
127. Lumen N, Monstrey S, Goessaert AS, et al. Urethroplasty for strictures after phallic reconstruction: a single-institution experience. Eur Urol 2011;60(1): 150–8.
128. Thum HW, Hoebeke P, Gooren LJ. Sex reassignment of transsexual people from a gynecologist's and urologist's perspective. Acta Obstet Gynecol Scand 2015; 94:563–7.
129. Selvaggi G, Hoebeke P, Ceulemans P, et al. Scrotal reconstruction in female-to-male transsexuals a novel scrotoplasty. Plast Reconstr Surg 2009;123(6): 1710–8.
130. Djordjevic ML, Bizic M, Stanojevic D, et al. Urethral lengthening in metoidioplasty (female-to-male sex reassignment surgery) by combined buccal mucosa graft and labia minora flap. Urology 2009;74(2):349–53.
131. Murad MH, Elamin MB, Garcia MZ, et al. Hormonal therapy and sex reassignment: a systematic review and meta-analysis of quality of life and psychosocial outcomes. Clin Endocrinol (Oxf) 2010. http://dx.doi.org/10.1111/j.1365-2265. 2009.03625.x.
132. White Hughto JM, Reisner SL. A systematic review of the effects of hormone therapy on psychological functioning and quality of life in transgender individuals. Transgend Health 2016;1(1):21–31.
133. Colizzi M, Costa R, Todarello O. Transsexual patients' psychiatric comorbidity and positive effect of cross-sex hormonal treatment on mental health: results from a longitudinal study. Psychoneuroendocrinology 2014;39:65–73.
134. Heylens G, Verroken C, De Cock S, et al. Effects of different steps in gender reassignment therapy on psychopathology: a prospective study of persons with a gender identity disorder. J Sex Med 2014;11(1):119–26.
135. Manieri C, Castellano E, Crespi C, et al. Medical treatment of subjects with gender identity disorder: the experience in an Italian public health center. Int J Transgend 2014;15(2):53–65.
136. Carmel TC, Erickson-Schroth L. Mental health and the transgender population. Psychiatr Ann 2016;46(6):346–9.
137. de Vries ALC, McGuire JK, Steensma TD, et al. Young adult psychological outcome after puberty suppression and gender reassignment. Pediatrics 2014;134(4):696–704.
138. Dhejne C, Oberg K, Arver S, et al. An analysis of all applications for sex reassignment surgery in Sweden, 1960–2010: prevalence, incidence, and regrets. Arch Sex Behav 2014;43:1535–45.
139. Michel A, Ansseau M, Legros JJ, et al. The transsexual: what about the future? Eur Psychiatry 2002;17(6):353–62.
140. Pfafflin F, Junge A. Sex reassignment. Thirty years of international follow-up studies after SRS: a comprehensive review. Dusseldorf (Germany): Symposion Publishing; 1998.

# Hormonal and Surgical Treatment Options for Transgender Women and Transfeminine Spectrum Persons

Linda M. Wesp, MSN, FNP-C[a],*, Madeline B. Deutsch, MD, MPH[b]

## KEYWORDS

- Transgender • Feminizing hormones • Feminizing surgery • Gender-affirming care
- Cross-sex hormones

## KEY POINTS

- Feminizing hormone therapy includes treatment with antiandrogens and estrogen supplementation in an individualized manner based on patient goals and health needs.
- Hormone therapy leads to development of feminine secondary sex characteristics and minimization of masculine characteristics; results vary greatly based on age, physiology and individual genetics.
- Surgical options may be limited owing to economic and structural barriers. Types of surgery pursued vary based on patient goals and status of hormone therapy.
- Hormone and surgical therapies improve quality of life and mental health in transgender people with minimal adverse effects.
- Ongoing longitudinal research is crucial to improve understanding about specific risks of feminizing hormone therapy and improve surgical outcomes.

## INTRODUCTION

Many (but not all) transgender individuals who identify on the female gender spectrum will seek medical interventions to affirm their gender. Health care providers trained in transgender care can prescribe feminizing hormone regimens, and surgeons trained in gender-affirming procedures can perform a variety of surgeries

Disclosures: Dr M.B. Deutsch is a co-principal investigator on a study that uses donated study drug from Gilead.
Funding Sources: None.
[a] College of Nursing, University of Wisconsin-Milwaukee, 1921 E. Hartford Avenue, Milwaukee, WI 53211, USA; [b] Department of Family & Community Medicine, Center of Excellence for Transgender Health, University of California - San Francisco, 2356 Sutter Street, 3rd Floor, San Francisco, CA 94143, USA
* Corresponding author. College of Nursing, University of Wisconsin-Milwaukee, PO Box 413, Milwaukee, WI 53201.
E-mail address: lmwesp@uwm.edu

Psychiatr Clin N Am 40 (2017) 99–111
http://dx.doi.org/10.1016/j.psc.2016.10.006
0193-953X/17/© 2016 Elsevier Inc. All rights reserved.

| Abbreviation | |
|---|---|
| WPATH | World Professional Association for Transgender Health |

to achieve feminization of the body. A gender-affirming and patient-centered model of care considers the individual goals and informed consent as central to the overall treatment plan. As such, some individuals pursue hormonal and/or surgical procedures with some degree of variation depending on multiple individual factors, in consultation with the health care team. Many, but not all, transgender women and transfeminine-spectrum people begin estrogen plus antiandrogen hormone therapy simultaneously to reduce masculine secondary sex characteristics and induce the development of feminine secondary sex characteristics. An increasing number of people, in part owing to improved insurance coverage, will seek a variety of surgeries, including facial feminization, breast augmentation, and genital affirmation surgery. This article provides an overview of current hormonal and surgical options for transfeminine individuals, based on a synthesis of best practice guidelines, a growing body of evidence, and the clinical experience of the authors who have collectively worked with transgender patients for 24 years.

### Gender-Affirming Care

When seeking consultation for hormones and surgery, it is crucial that each individual's gender identity is affirmed.[1,2] In addition to basic components such as use of one's chosen name and pronoun, gender affirmation in health care encounters includes discussing specific goals, which vary from patient to patient and may not fit into traditional gender binary expectations. Medical and behavioral health providers are responsible for an ongoing process of informed consent. For hormonal options, discussions include exploring all possible changes and uncertainty of precise outcomes, level of permanency, risk of adverse events, and when to expect onset and maximum effect of hormones. For surgical options, counseling includes preoperative and postoperative care planning with an interdisciplinary health care team[3] and a detailed conversation with the surgeon about the procedure itself, including a discussion of risks and possible complications.

Some individuals presenting for hormone care may request a mix of masculine and feminine characteristics, others may seek a slower transition, and still others may present with goals that may not be realistic given the way hormones work in the body. For example, it is unlikely that feminizing hormone regimen alone will eliminate all unwanted facial hair, and therefore electrolysis or laser hair removal is often required. Alternatively, feminizing hormone therapy, even at low doses, will almost always lead to some breast development as well as loss of erectile function; therefore, these realities have to be taken into consideration. Furthermore, the same medication and dose can have very different effects from person to person, depending on concurrent medications, physiology, and genetics. Best practice guidelines such as Center of Excellence for Transgender Health Guidelines for Primary and Gender-Affirming Care of Transgender and Gender Nonbinary People,[4] World Professional Association for Transgender Health (WPATH) Standards of Care, 7th Version,[5] and Endocrine Society Clinical Practice Guidelines[6] can guide clinical practice. However, treatments are individualized based on an informed discussion about long-term risks, realistic expectations, and the patient's goals. The recommended hormone dosages discussed in this article may be started at lower amounts and increased more slowly, titrating to the desired effect.

## HORMONE THERAPY

Maximum development of female secondary sex characteristics and minimization of male secondary sex characteristics will be achieved when testosterone levels are lowered into the female physiologic range and physiologic doses of estrogen are administered. Long-term data are lacking; however, anecdotal sources suggest that maximal feminization may occur within 2 to 5 years of uninterrupted therapy.[6] For individuals who retain their gonads, maximum feminization is achieved by combining an androgen blocker with an estrogen. Although all medications used for feminizing hormone therapy are approved by the Food and Drug Administration for use in cisgender women, their use in transgender women is off-label and may be at higher doses.

This overview focuses on treatments available for adults who have undergone full puberty. However, an increasing number of transgender and gender nonconforming adolescents are receiving gender-affirming care that includes puberty blockade and introduction of cross-sex hormones before the completion of the undesired puberty. These individuals will have fewer undesired secondary sex characteristics, and will likely present to adult providers on maintenance doses of antiandrogens plus estrogen. For more detailed information on gender-affirming care for transgender adolescents, interested readers may refer to the Center of Excellence for Transgender Health Guidelines for Primary and Gender-Affirming Care of Transgender and Gender Nonbinary People[4] and WPATH Standards of Care, 7th Version.[5]

### Effects of Feminizing Hormone Therapy

Changes that can be expected with hormone therapy include breast development, a redistribution of facial and body subcutaneous fat, reduction of muscle mass, reduction of body hair quantity and thickness (less so for facial hair), change in sweat and odor patterns, and slowing or reversal of scalp hair loss. Genital and reproductive effects include reduction in erectile function, reduced or absent sperm count and ejaculatory fluid, and reduced testicular size. Changes in libido or sexual desire after initiation of feminizing hormone therapy may also occur. Prospective studies are lacking to determine the specific relationship to hormone levels and/or surgical status. One retrospective cross-sectional study of transgender women (n = 214) on hormone therapy found that 22.1% self-reported currently experiencing hypoactive sexual desire disorder. The researchers reported that type of hormones, duration of hormone treatment, and satisfaction with hormone therapy were not associated with hypoactive sexual desire disorder. The majority of people in the study (64.8%) had undergone sexual reassignment surgery and, among these, there was a self-reported increase in spontaneous sexual desire after the surgery.[7]

Feminizing hormone therapy may also bring about changes in mood. Estrogen and progesterone are likely associated with mental health conditions in cisgender populations, such as premenstrual dysphoric disorder, but studies exploring relationships between hormone levels and mental health conditions in transgender women are lacking. One study from Spain (n − 187) measured social anxiety using the Social Anxiety and Depression Scale, as well as current symptoms of anxiety and depression with the Hospital Anxiety and Depression Scale[8] comparing transgender people who were taking hormone therapy with those who were on a waiting list to begin hormone therapy. People on hormones actually had lower anxiety/depression scores and improved social functioning, compared with those who were waiting to begin hormones. In general, mental health concerns before and after the initiation of hormones should be considered in context of the patient's individual symptoms and history, taking into consideration that mood may be impacted positively or negatively.

Table 1 provides an overview of feminization effects. Times to expected onset and maximum effect are estimations based on anecdotal experience and various guidelines.[5,6] As mentioned, some masculine characteristics are not reversible with feminizing hormone therapy alone. Feminizing hormone therapy does not eliminate facial and body hair, change skeletal bone shape or height, or change the pitch of the voice. Once testosterone has impacted these elements during puberty, they are not reversed by feminization therapy and require interventions such as electrolysis or laser hair removal, plastic surgery, or voice/speech therapy.

## Estrogens

Estrogens lead to the development of female secondary sex characteristics throughout the body, namely breast development, body fat redistribution, and skin softening. Although used off-label in gender-affirming care, estrogen therapy is composed of Food and Drug Administration–approved 17-beta estradiol (or more simply, estradiol). Estradiol is a bioidentical hormone that has "exactly the same chemical and molecular structure as hormones that are produced in the human body."[9] Estradiol in the context of gender-affirming care is most commonly administered orally, by

**Table 1**
**Effects of feminizing hormone therapy**

| Effect | Time to Expected Onset (mo) | Time to Expected Maximum Effect[a] | Permanency if Estrogen Stopped |
|---|---|---|---|
| Breast growth | 3–6 | 2–3 y | Permanent |
| Thinning of body and facial hair | 6–12 | >3 y | Reversible |
| Slowing of male pattern scalp balding | 1–2 | 1–2 y | Reversible |
| Softening of skin/decreased oiliness | 3–6 | Unknown | Reversible |
| Body fat redistribution | 3–6 | 2–5 y | Reversible |
| Decreased muscle mass/strength | 3–6 | 1–2 y | Reversible |
| Decreased libido | 1–3 | 1–2 y | Reversible |
| Decreased spontaneous/morning erections | 1–3 | 3–6 mo | Reversible |
| Decreased erectile firmness and ejaculation | 1–3 | Variable | Reversible |
| Decreased sperm production/fertility | Variable | Variable | Reversible or permanent[b] |
| Decreased testicular volume | 3–6 | 2–3 y | Unknown |

[a] Time at which further changes are unlikely at maximum maintained dose. Maximum effects vary widely depending on genetics, body habitus, age, and status of gonad removal. Generally, older individuals with intact gonads may have fewer feminization effects overall.

[b] Further research is needed; however, all patients beginning estrogen therapy should be counseled on sperm preservation options before initiation of therapy owing to likely permanent impact on sperm quality.

*Adapted from* Hembree WC, Cohen-Kettenis P, Delemarre-van de Waal HA, et al. Endocrine treatment of transsexual persons: an endocrine society clinical practice guideline. J Clin Endocrinol Metab 2009;94:3132–54.

transdermal patch, or by injection. Ethinyl estradiol (found in combined oral contraceptives) is not used, and conjugated equine estrogens are not recommended owing to concerns about increased thrombogenicity and cardiovascular risk.[10-12] **Table 2** provides an overview of recommended 17-beta estradiol formulations.

Owing to the significant thrombogenic risk of estrogens in the setting of tobacco use, tobacco cessation counseling is offered regularly for those beginning estrogen therapy. Data from studies in postmenopausal cisgender women suggest that oral estrogen therapy may be associated with increased risk for thrombosis compared with a transdermal route, although the absolute difference in risk is likely small.[13] Transdermal estradiol and possibly sublingual administration of micronized oral estradiol tablets may mitigate thromboembolic risk in patients at higher risk via avoidance of first-pass hepatic metabolism.[14]

### Antiandrogens

The current approach to feminization therapy involves medications that block androgens along with estrogen therapy at physiologic doses. Clinicians no longer use excessive estrogen, which, before the use of antiandrogens, was administered to inhibit endogenous testosterone production via suppression of gonadotropins and to induce feminizing secondary sex characteristics. Excessive estrogen doses are avoided to minimize cardiovascular and thromboembolism risks as well as estrogenic side effects such as migraines.

Spironolactone, an orally administered, potassium-sparing diuretic is the most commonly used androgen blocker in the United States, and is an effective component

**Table 2**
**Options for 17-beta estradiol**

| Formulation | Initial Dose | Maximum Dose | Comments |
|---|---|---|---|
| Transdermal | 100 μg | 400 μg | Patches only come as 100 μg, so if maximum dose is required, more than 1 patch must be worn. Frequency of patch change is brand/product dependent, but usually once per week. |
| Oral/sublingual | 2–4 mg/d | 8 mg/d | May be divided into twice daily dosing. Sublingual absorption usually takes 10–15 min. |
| Estradiol valerate IM | 20 mg intramuscularly every 2 wk | 40 mg intramuscularly every 2 wk | Concentration may be 20 mg/mL or 40 mg/mL. Vial sizes vary. May divide dose into weekly injections to avoid cyclical symptoms. |
| Estradiol cypionate IM | 2.5 mg intramuscularly every 2 wk | 5 mg IM every 2 wk | Concentration usually 5 mg/mL. |

of transitioning regimens.[15] Owing to its relatively effract, particularly among experiences transsexual frequency of urination or orthostatic symptoms. Patients taking spironolactone should undergo periodic monitoring of renal function and potassium, although anecdotally renal complications are rare. Another choice for antiandrogens are oral 5 alpha reductase inhibitors finasteride and dutasteride, which block conversion of testosterone to the potent androgen dihydrotestosterone[16] and may be a good choice for patients who are unable to take spironolactone owing to contraindications or drug–drug interactions. Some clinicians use a low dose of finasteride in addition to spironolactone to treat male pattern baldness. **Table 3** summarizes antiandrogen medication dosing.

Spironolactone or 5-alpha reductase inhibitors may also be used in lower doses alone (ie, without estrogen) for individuals who desire minimal or slower transition. In the absence of estrogen replacement, androgen blockade may lead to unpleasant symptoms of hot flashes and low mood or energy.[4] Additionally, long-term suppression of androgens without any hormone replacement raises concern for osteopenia; full androgen blockade without hormone replacement in men who have undergone treatment for prostate cancer has been related to bone loss.[17] Therefore, although short-term androgen suppression is a temporary option for individuals who desire a slower transition, long-term and complete androgen suppression without estrogen supplementation is not recommended, owing to the potential risk for bone loss.[4]

### Progestagens

The role of progestagens in feminizing hormone therapy is unclear. Some providers and patients believe progestagens may enhance breast development, mood, or libido; however, evidence is lacking and some may experience negative mood effects.[18] The primary concern with the combined use of progestagens and estrogens is an increased risk of cardiovascular events and breast cancer reported in studies of postmenopausal women; however, no studies have been conducted in transgender women. Common preparations for feminizing regimens include micronized progesterone 100 to 200 mg/d or medroxyprogesterone 5 to 10 mg/d. Cyproterone acetate (not available in the United States) is a progestational compound widely used as an androgen blocker in Europe.[19]

### Hormone Management and Monitoring

The initial medication and dose should be based on patient goals, with consideration given to coexisting health conditions and risk factors. Weak evidence suggests that initiating estradiol at lower doses, with upward titration over time and delayed initiation of antiandrogens, may result in enhanced breast development,[20] an approach that is

| Table 3 Recommended antiandrogen dose | | | |
|---|---|---|---|
| Drug | Initial Dose (mg/d) | Maximum Dose (mg/d) | Comments |
| Spironolactone | 100 | 400 | Usually divided into twice daily dosing. Pills come in 25, 50, or 100 mg doses and can be titrated up as tolerated. Taking earlier in day may prevent urinary frequency during night. |
| Finasteride | 1 | 5 | Pills come in 1 or 5 mg. |
| Dutasteride | 0.5 | 0.5 | — |

consistent with the management of children with delayed puberty. In all cases, the regimen and titration schedule should be in part guided by patient preference, and any assessment of risks of treatment should be considered in the context of the known benefits of hormone therapy.[21]

Once any therapy is initiated at any dose, monitoring is composed of both laboratory blood testing and patient follow-up visits. Blood tests monitor for adverse outcomes as well as target serum hormone levels, which should be maintained within the female physiologic level. The frequency of blood testing may be impacted by availability of resources or insurance factors. Some providers choose to focus on safety monitoring only (ie, serum potassium and renal function when using spironolactone), use clinical visits to monitor clinical progress, and check hormone levels only if clinical goals are not being reached. Conversely, the Endocrine Society Clinical Practice Guidelines recommend blood monitoring of hormone levels every 3 months for the first year and then once or twice yearly.[6] A prospective study of transgender women taking a 4 mg/d divided dose of oral estradiol or 100 μg transdermal estradiol, plus a 100 to 200 mg/d divided dose of spironolactone found that total testosterone levels remained increased in 33% at 6 months,[22] suggesting that monitoring of hormone levels to guide therapy adjustments within the first year may be useful to maximize therapy. Additionally, because suppression of testosterone is of particular concern in ensuring maximal feminization, the calculation of bioavailable testosterone in transgender women may be of value. Specifically, exogenous estrogens (especially oral) may be associated with increased levels of sex hormone–binding globulin; such increases can vary from person to person and across regimens. Therefore, in cases of patient concern or persistent virilized features in the presence of a female-range total testosterone, calculation of the bioavailable testosterone may help to fine tune hormone regimens for optimal effect. Overall, evidence is lacking to guide laboratory monitoring, and most clinicians use a combination of clinical monitoring and laboratory tests to guide dose titration.

Once individuals reach a maintenance phase, often after 1 year of stable dose therapy, clinical visits and laboratory monitoring can take place annually unless otherwise indicated by coexisting conditions or clinical symptoms. Frequency may increase owing to significant changes in health status, such as onset of diabetes or a thyroid disorder, substantial weight changes, subjective or objective evidence of virilization, or new symptoms potentially precipitated or exacerbated by hormone imbalances such as hot flashes or migraines. An increased frequency of office visits may also be useful for patients with complex psychosocial situations to allow for the provision of ancillary or wraparound services. Screening prolactin monitoring is of questionable value, because the current standard of care for an incidentally detected and asymptomatic prolactinoma is observation only, unless symptoms develop such as headaches, peripheral vision loss, or galactorrhea.[23] Common laboratory monitoring is summarized in **Table 4**.

Both hormones and genital surgery have an impact on future fertility. Estrogen has an unknown effect on spermatogenesis and penile function,[24] and surgical removal of the testes results in permanent sterility. Therefore, fertility counseling before hormone therapy and surgery are paramount to discuss the options of sperm cryopreservation, surgical sperm extraction, or testicular tissue cryopreservation.[25] Many individuals face constraints, however, because these procedures may not be covered by insurance and are often cost prohibitive. Alternatively, some transgender women do still produce sperm at various stages of feminization, and reproductive counseling should also include conversations about unplanned pregnancy if they are engaging in sexual activity that could result in pregnancy.

**Table 4**
**Common laboratory monitoring for feminizing hormone therapy**

| | Comments | Baseline | Quarterly During First Year of Therapy | Yearly | As Needed Based on Medical History and Clinician Discretion |
|---|---|---|---|---|---|
| BUN/Cr/K$^+$ | Used to monitor for adverse effects of spironolactone. | X | X | X | X |
| Estradiol | — | — | X | — | X |
| Total testosterone | Some clinicians may also monitor bioavailable testosterone | — | X | — | X |
| Lipids | — | — | — | — | X |
| Hemoglobin A1c or glucose | — | — | — | — | X |
| Prolactin | — | — | — | — | X |

*Abbreviations:* BUN, blood urea nitrogen; Cr, creatinine.

*Adapted from* Center of Excellence for Transgender Health, Department of Family and Community Medicine, University of California San Francisco. Guidelines for the primary and gender-affirming care of transgender and gender nonbinary people, 2nd edition. 2016. Updated Deutsch MB, ed. 2016. Available at: http://www.transhealth.ucsf.edu/trans?page=guidelines-feminizing-therapy. Accessed July 12, 2016; with permission.

## SURGICAL OPTIONS

A variety of surgical procedures is available for gender affirmation and is summarized in **Table 5**. Access to surgery has increased owing to the growing elimination of transgender exclusions in health care insurance, including some state Medicaid programs and federal Medicare policies.[26,27] However, many still face prohibitive deductibles or other out-of-pocket costs, and an elimination of exclusion does not always equate to coverage for a procedure. The number of surgeons with experience and training in gender-affirming procedures are limited, and many major US cities lack any surgical capacity. Many patients endure long waiting lists and must travel significant distances. The WPATH Standards of Care, 7th Version, describes readiness and eligibility criteria for gender-affirming chest and genital procedures[5] (see **Table 5**). These criteria are often referenced by insurance companies when determining eligibility for coverage. Many patients may lack access to qualified mental health providers within their insurance networks to support them in preparing for surgery and to conduct the required assessments. In addition to the assessment and readiness criteria described by WPATH, further psychosocial and educational support is often required to prepare for and navigate the complexities of preoperative planning and postoperative self-care.[3] The reality of which surgical options are obtainable and the level of support available to navigate the procedures and healing, thus depends on a variety of structural and economic factors.

| Table 5<br>Gender-affirming surgeries and WPATH SOCv7 criteria | | |
|---|---|---|
| Procedure and<br>SOCv7 Criteria | Description | Comments |
| Orchiectomy[a,b] | Removal of testicles | Scrotal skin is not removed. May be done alone or simultaneously with vaginoplasty. |
| Vaginoplasty[a,b] | Creation of neovagina, clitoris; rerouting of urethra. May also include labiaplasty, which is creation of labia from scrotal skin. | Most common procedure is penile inversion technique. Prostate is left in place anterior to neovagina. |
| Breast augmentation[a,c] | Surgical placement of bilateral breast implants | Most often implants contain silicone. |
| Facial feminization[d] | Plastic surgery the forehead, nose, cheeks, lips, chin, and/or jawline. | Varies by individual and surgeon, may also include hair transplantation. |
| Reduction thyroid chondroplasty[d] | Reduction of thyroid cartilage | Decreases prominence of the "Adam's apple" |

*Abbreviation:* WPATH SOCv7, World Professional Association for Transgender Health Standards of Care, 7th Version.
[a] Persistent, well-documented gender dysphoria and the capacity to make a fully informed decision to consent for treatment.
[b] Two letters of referral from qualified mental health professionals and 12 months of continuous hormone therapy as appropriate to patient gender goals.
[c] Feminizing hormone therapy for a minimum of 12 months before breast augmentation surgery is recommended to best fit the feminized chest contour.
[d] No criteria offered.
*From* Coleman E, Bockting W, Botzer M, et al. Standards of care for the health of transsexual, transgender, and gender nonconforming people, 7th version. Int J Transgend 2012;13:227; with permission.

### Genital Procedures

Genital affirmation surgeries include orchiectomy (removal of testicles), vaginoplasty (creation of a vagina), and labiaplasty (creation of labia). Orchiectomy may be performed alone or in conjunction with a vaginoplasty procedure. Antiandrogen medication can be discontinued after orchiectomy.

The most commonly performed procedure for vaginoplasty is known as the penile inversion technique.[28,29] Before surgery, most patients require electrolysis or laser hair removal along the penile shaft, scrotum, and perineum to prevent hair growth inside the neovagina (the term used to describe a surgically constructed vagina in a transgender woman). Vaginoplasty involves the creation of a neovaginal cavity from scrotal and penile skin, repositioning of the urethra, and the creation of clitoral/intravaginal sensate tissue from the glans penis,[30,31] although specific techniques vary widely from surgeon to surgeon. To prevent vaginal stenosis, regular dilation is required postoperatively using dilators. Healing can take up to 6 to 8 weeks, at which time vaginal intercourse can begin if desired.[29] Complications include vaginal stenosis and fistulas.[28] During this procedure, the prostate remains anteriorly to the neovagina. Labiaplasty is often performed at the time of vaginoplasty, and includes the creation of labia, most commonly using scrotal skin. Some surgeons recommend delayed [illegible] as a second procedure, and some patients may choose to pursue additional labiaplasty surgeries at a later time.[29]

### Breast Augmentation

Breast growth may be unsatisfactory with hormonal therapy alone; therefore, some individuals pursue augmentation mammoplasty using saline or silicone implants. The location of the implant varies based on individual body shape and amount of growth on hormones.[29] To best fit the feminized chest contour, surgeons generally recommend at least 1 year on hormone therapy before undergoing breast augmentation surgery.

### Face, Head, and Neck Procedures

Some individuals may pursue face, head, and neck procedures for gender affirmation. Facial feminization is a term used to broadly describe a variety of plastic surgery techniques altering the bony structures of the forehead, nose, cheeks, lips, chin, and/or jawline. Procedures may also include hair transplantation to address androgenic alopecia and other hair loss. A reduction thyrochondroplasty, or "tracheal shave," is a specific procedure to reduce the thyroid cartilage to decrease the prominent appearance of the "Adam's apple." Feminizing speech therapy has been shown to be effective in improving self-image and quality of life; surgical procedures to modify vocal pitch are uncommon but may have a role after an optimal course of speech therapy.[4]

## OUTCOMES

A systematic review found 3 prospective cohort studies that measured exposure to hormones and subsequent changes in mental health and quality-of-life outcomes, using a wide variety of psychometrically valid and reliable self-report scales.[21] The review suggested that transgender women (n = 180) report a significant increase in general quality of life after initiating hormone therapy, but that higher quality evidence, such as longitudinal controlled trials, are needed. A systematic review of 28 mostly observational studies enrolling a total of 1093 transgender women who received both hormones and surgery found evidence that these gender affirmation interventions were associated with decreased gender dysphoria, improved quality of life, and improved psychological symptoms on self-report.[32] Studies exploring self-reported outcomes after vaginoplasty surgery have also found improved global functioning, sexual functioning, family and interpersonal relationships, body image, and quality of life.[33,34] A cost-effectiveness study found a savings of $8655 per quality-adjusted life-year when gender-affirming procedures are covered by insurance.[35]

Long-term data on risks of hormone therapy are lacking in the United States. Longitudinal follow-up studies in Europe suggest that feminizing hormone therapy may be associated with an increased incidence of cardiovascular disease and osteoporosis, but did not control for risk factors such as tobacco use and have not that demonstrated hormone therapy causes greater mortality.[36,37] Individuals who have undergone gonadectomy should remain on estrogen therapy until at least age 50 to prevent osteoporosis. Data on breast,[38] prostate,[39] and testicular[40] cancers are limited, but suggest that transgender women who have these organs can still get cancer, although those on feminizing hormone therapy are likely at a lesser risk than cisgender people for testicular and prostate cancers owing to androgen blockade. Further longitudinal research is necessary draw specific conclusions about the exact levels of risk for people on feminizing hormone therapy, compared with those not on hormones. Consideration and management of cardiovascular disease, bone disease, and cancer are an ongoing component of primary care for transgender individuals who receive hormone or surgical interventions, and future research specific to transgender populations will continue to inform evidence-based care.

## SUMMARY

Transgender people have a variety of hormonal and surgical options available for gender affirmation. Decisions about which options to pursue involve collaboration with knowledgeable health care providers and an ongoing process of informed consent, taking into consideration patient goals and individual factors. Economic and social factors will also impact the choices available; therefore, ongoing policy and advocacy work is needed to equalize opportunities. Evidence suggests that those who pursue feminization with hormones and/or surgery experience reduced gender dysphoria as well as improvements in quality of life, decreased depression and anxiety, and overall long-term health, and that these interventions are cost effective. Future research will improve understanding about specific risks of feminizing hormone therapy and improve surgical outcomes.

## REFERENCES

1. Sevelius JM. Gender affirmation: a framework for conceptualizing risk behavior among transgender women of color. Sex Roles 2013;68(11–12):675–89.
2. Bockting W, Coleman E, Deutsch MB, et al. Adult development and quality of life of transgender and gender nonconforming people. Curr Opin Endocrinol Diabetes Obes 2016;23:188–97.
3. Deutsch MB. Gender affirming surgeries in the era of insurance coverage: developing a framework for psychosocial support and care navigation in the perioperative period. J Health Care Poor Underserved 2016;27:1–6.
4. Center of Excellence for Transgender Health, Department of Family and Community Medicine, University of California San Francisco. Guidelines for the primary and gender-affirming care of transgender and gender nonbinary people, 2nd edition. Updated Deutsch, MB, ed. 2016. 2016. Available at: www.transhealth.ucsf.edu/guidelines. Accessed July 12, 2016.
5. Coleman E, Bockting W, Botzer M, et al. Standards of care for the health of transsexual, transgender, and gender nonconforming people, 7th version. Int J Transgend 2012;13:165–232.
6. Hembree WC, Cohen-Kettenis P, Delemarre-van de Waal HA, et al. Endocrine treatment of transsexual persons: an endocrine society clinical practice guideline. J Clin Endocrinol Metab 2009;94(9):3132–54.
7. Wierckx K, Elaut E, Van Hoorde B, et al. Sexual desire in trans persons: associations with sex reassignment treatment. Journal of Sexual Medicine 2014;11(1):107–18.
8. Gomez-Gil E, Zubiaurre-Elorza L, Esteva I, et al. Hormone-treated transsexuals report less social distress, anxiety and depression. Psychoneuroendocrinology 2012;37(5):662–70.
9. The Endocrine Society. Position statements of the endocrine society: bioidentical hormones. 2009. Available at: https://www.endocrine.org/advocacy-and-outreach/position-statements. Accessed August 22, 2016.
10. Shifren JL, Rifai N, Desindes S, et al. A comparison of the short-term effects of oral conjugated equine estrogens versus transdermal estradiol on C-reactive protein, other serum markers of inflammation, and other hepatic proteins in naturally menopausal women. J Clin Endocrinol Metab 2008;93(5):1702–10.

11. Lacut K, Oger E, Mottier D, et al. Differential effects of oral conjugated equine estrogen and transdermal estrogen on atherosclerotic vascular disease risk markers and endothelial function in healthy postmenopausal women. Hum Reprod 2006;21(10):2715–20.

12. Hugon-Rodin J, Gompel A, Plu-Bureau G. Epidemiology of hormonal contraceptives-related venous thromboembolism. Eur J Endocrinol 2014;171(6):R221–30.

13. Mohammed K, Abu Dabrh AM, Benkhadra K, et al. Oral vs transdermal estrogen therapy and vascular events: a systematic review and meta-analysis. J Clin Endocrinol Metab 2015;100(11):4012–20.

14. Price TM, Blauer KL, Hansen M, et al. Single-dose pharmacokinetics of sublingual versus oral administration of micronized 17 beta-estradiol. Obstet Gynecol 1997;89(3):340–5.

15. Prior JC, Vigna YM, Watson D. Spironolactone with physiological female steroids for presurgical therapy of male-to-female transsexualism. Arch Sex Behav 1989; 18(1):49–57.

16. Rittmaster RS. 5alpha-reductase inhibitors. J Androl 1997;18(6):582–7.

17. Bienz M, Saad F. Androgen-deprivation therapy and bone loss in prostate cancer patients: a clinical review. Bonekey Rep 2015;4:716.

18. Wierckx K, Gooren L, T'Sjoen G. Clinical review: breast development in trans women receiving cross-sex hormones. J Sex Med 2014;11(5):1240–7.

19. Gooren LJ. Management of female-to-male transgender persons: medical and surgical management, life expectancy. Curr Opin Endocrinol Diabetes Obes 2014;21(3):233–8.

20. Seal LJ, Franklin S, Richards C, et al. Predictive markers for mammoplasty and a comparison of side effect profiles in transwomen taking various hormonal regimens. J Clin Endocrinol Metab 2012;97(12):4422–8.

21. White Hughto JM, Reisner SL. A systematic review of the effects of hormone therapy on psychological functioning and quality of life in transgender individuals. Transgender Health 2016;1(1):21–31.

22. Deutsch MB, Bhakri V, Kubicek K. Effects of cross-sex hormone treatment on transgender women and men. Obstet Gynecol 2015;125(3):605–10.

23. Freda PU, Beckers AM, Katznelson L, et al. Pituitary incidentaloma: an endocrine society clinical practice guideline. J Clin Endocrinol Metab 2011;96(4):894–904.

24. Schulster M, Bernie AM, Ramasamy R. The role of estradiol in male reproductive function. Asian J Androl 2016;18(3):435–40.

25. De Roo C, Tilleman K, T'Sjoen G, et al. Fertility options in transgender people. Int Rev Psychiatry 2016;28(1):112–9.

26. Green J. Transsexual surgery may be covered by medicare. LGBT Health 2014; 1(4):256–8.

27. National Center for Transgender Equality. Know your rights: Medicare. 2014. Available at: http://www.transequality.org/know-your-rights/medicare. Accessed August 22, 2016.

28. Horbach SE, Bouman MB, Smit JM, et al. Outcome of vaginoplasty in male-to-female transgenders: a systematic review of surgical techniques. J Sex Med 2015;12(6):1499–512.

29. Schechter LS. Gender confirmation surgery: an update for the primary care provider. Transgender Health 2016;1(1):32–40.

30. Kanhai RC. Sensate vagina pedicled-spot for male-to-female transsexuals: the experience in the first 50 patients. Aesthetic Plast Surg 2016;40(2):284–7.

31. Leclere FM, Casoli V, Baudet J, et al. Description of the Baudet surgical technique and introduction of a systematic method for training surgeons to perform

male-to-female sex reassignment surgery. Aesthetic Plast Surg 2015;39(6): 927–34.

32. Murad MH, Elamin MB, Garcia MZ, et al. Hormonal therapy and sex reassignment: a systematic review and meta-analysis of quality of life and psychosocial outcomes. Clin Endocrinol (Oxf) 2010;72(2):214–31.

33. Michel A, Ansseau M, Legros JJ, et al. The transsexual: what about the future? Eur Psychiatry 2002;17(6):353–62.

34. Lawrence AA. Factors associated with satisfaction or regret following male-to-female sex reassignment surgery. Arch Sex Behav 2003;32(4):299–315.

35. Padula WV, Heru S, Campbell JD. Societal implications of health insurance coverage for medically necessary services in the U.S. transgender population: a cost-effectiveness analysis. J Gen Intern Med 2016;31(4):394–401.

36. Gooren LJ, Giltay EJ, Bunck MC. Long-term treatment of transsexuals with cross-sex hormones: extensive personal experience. J Clin Endocrinol Metab 2008; 93(1):19–25.

37. Wierckx K, Mueller S, Weyers S, et al. Long-term evaluation of cross-sex hormone treatment in transsexual persons. J Sex Med 2012;9(10):2641–51.

38. Brown GR, Jones KT. Incidence of breast cancer in a cohort of 5,135 transgender veterans. Breast Cancer Res Treat 2015;149(1):191–8.

39. Miksad RA, Bubley G, Church P, et al. Prostate cancer in a transgender woman 41 years after initiation of feminization. JAMA 2006;296(19):2316–7.

40. Wolf-Gould CS, Wolf-Gould CH. A transgender woman with testicular cancer: a new twist on an old problem. LGBT Health 2015;3(1):90–5.

# Working Toward Family Attunement

## Family Therapy with Transgender and Gender-Nonconforming Children and Adolescents

Deborah Coolhart, PhD, LMFT*, Daran L. Shipman, MA, LMFT

## KEYWORDS

- Transgender • Gender nonconforming • Youth • Family • Therapy
- Gender affirmative • Support

## KEY POINTS

- Gender-affirmative family therapy assumes that transgender and gender-nonconforming (TGNC) identities are natural variations of humanity that should be normalized and affirmed.
- Family therapy first seeks to assess and increase family members' attunement to the TGNC child's gender expression.
- Clinicians provide safety for the TGNC youth by working with parents and other family members to better support their child and by creating a gender-affirming environment in therapy.
- When the family is ready, options for gender expression/transition are explored and supported in therapy.
- As needed, the clinician advocates for the TGNC youth in school and other settings and supports families through the readiness process for social and medical gender transition.

*The Suarez family: "Steven," a 7 year old who was assigned a male gender at birth, has been secretly dressing in his mother's clothing and getting into her makeup. On discovering her child's behavior, Steven's mother reacted with shock and disapproval, which resulted in Steven feeling ashamed and in tears. Steven's mother talked with him about why he was dressing in her clothing and Steven replied, "Because I want to be a girl. I don't like boy stuff and girl stuff is so much better." Steven's mother reprimanded him by telling him that his behavior is sinful and that he will go to hell if he does not stop. She sought the assistance of a family clinician to help Steven sort through his gender "confusion."*

Disclosure Statement: The authors have no conflict of interest and funding for this work.
Department of Marriage and Family Therapy, Syracuse University, 601 East Genesee Street, Peck Hall, Syracuse, NY 13202, USA
* Corresponding author.
*E-mail address:* dcoole@syr.edu

Psychiatr Clin N Am 40 (2017) 113–125
http://dx.doi.org/10.1016/j.psc.2016.10.002
0193-953X/17/© 2016 Elsevier Inc. All rights reserved.

*The Jackson family. "Julia," a 15 year old* who was assigned a female gender at birth, *has always hated wearing dresses and has been known as a tomboy, which her parents supported throughout Julie's childhood. As Julie has progressed into puberty, she has become increasingly uncomfortable with her body resulting in bouts of severe depression and self-harm. Her parents noticed her wearing more and more layers of baggy clothing and avoiding swimsuits. They noted they have been concerned about her body image and self-esteem and have been trying to assure Julie that she is a pretty girl who should be proud of her body. After several months of feeling nagged by her parents, Julie has disclosed to them that she is transgender and that she is really a boy. Her parents suspected that Julie might be a lesbian and were trying to come to terms with that; however, they have no real experience with or knowledge of transgender identities. They sought family therapy for assistance in figuring out what to do.*

As is seen from these case examples, the families of transgender and gender-nonconforming (TGNC) children and adolescents come to therapy at various stages of understanding and acceptance of their child's gender expressions. For these children to thrive, it is necessary to involve parents, and often other family members, in therapy. Family members often need to process their own feelings about the child's TGNC expressions and learn how to accept, support, and protect them in a society that is often hostile toward gender diverse people. This article presents a model for gender-affirmative family therapy with TGNC youth and their families, involving two stages: assessing and increasing family attunement (the family's level of understanding and peace about the TGNC identity), and exploring and supporting gender expression/transition options.

When families enter therapy already demonstrating a high level of understanding and support for the child's gender expression, they may spend less time in the first stage and may be ready to move into the second stage sooner, as is demonstrated in the case examples when as we follow them through the two stages of therapy.

## STAGE ONE: ASSESSING AND INCREASING FAMILY ATTUNEMENT

When beginning therapy with the family of a TGNC child, the first step is to assess how much support for and/or opposition to the gender expression is present in the family. The initial goal of family therapy is to help families more fully understand, accept, and learn to advocate for the TGNC child. The following section discusses this stage of therapy, beginning by defining gender-affirmative family therapy and family attunement. Strategies are then provided for structuring sessions and for working with family members, separately and together, in therapy.

### Moving Toward Attunement: Gender-Affirmative Family Therapy

The gender-affirmative clinician believes that gender-diverse expressions and identities do not constitute forms of pathology. They understand gender is not binary and instead exists on a spectrum with infinite expressions, all of which are normal variations of humanity. Gender-affirmative clinicians strive to destigmatize and normalize gender-nonconforming expressions,[1] helping TGNC children to live and express gender in ways that are most comfortable for the child.[2] Refer to **Box 1** for key terms and their definitions. Often for families presenting in therapy, what is most comfortable for the child is uncomfortable for the family and sometimes creates a considerable amount of distress for family members.[3] By supporting and validating parents in their emotional process, while at the same time creating safety and affirmation for the child, the gender-affirmative clinician seeks to help the family achieve attunement with their child's gender expression/identity. The term "attunement" means to reach a level of

---

**Box 1**
**Key terms**

Family Attunement: When a family experiences harmony, understanding, and peace regarding a family member's TGNC expression

Gender Affirmative: Therapeutic approach based on the belief that TGNC expressions are natural variations of humanity; seeking to normalize, validate, destigmatize, and support gender diversity

---

harmony, understanding, and peace about the child's gender expression/identity,[3] and to embrace the child's unique sense of gender. Note that this goes beyond tolerance, which typically leads to continued distress for youth, and toward celebration of their gendered selves. It is often helpful to be clear with parents about using a gender-affirmative approach in therapy during or before the initial session. Clinicians can explain that children only thrive in the face of being seen and valued for who they are and that not using a gender-affirmative approach could in fact cause more harm to their child.

### Why Is the Family Coming to Therapy and Who Will Attend Sessions?

There are several common presentations of families seeking therapy after the disclosure or discovery of their child's gender nonconformity. Many report first having challenging family conversations at home regarding gender, which then lead them to seek outside help. Some parents experience inner turmoil, guilt, or despair over why their child may be this way and want to know what to do about it. Parents may be angry, frustrated, disappointed, confused, and fearful. Sometimes the child is experiencing isolation and/or bullying and may be exhibiting self-harming behaviors, depressive or anxious symptoms, and sometimes suicidal ideations. Families may be seeking therapy because of the distress of their child, the distress of the parents, or sometimes it may be both. Therapy can be a place of refuge for all members of the family, where they can be honest and intimate, and where TGNC identities are nurtured.[4]

It is important to begin with the notion that the TGNC child may be no more in need of treatment than a gender-conforming child.[5] It may not be important for the child to enter treatment at all and instead the parents may enter treatment alone, at least initially. Creating a safe space for the youth is of utmost importance because it is extremely common for gender-nonconforming youth to have been exposed to many negative messages regarding their gender expression or identity. These messages may come from their external systems, such as peers, teachers, and church members. These messages may also come from within their family systems, where family members may be in distress and expressing views, thoughts, and feelings that are hurtful to the child. If this is the case, it is recommended that the child and other family members have separate sessions initially so therapy does not replicate a negative process, where the child is being harmed by their parents' expressions. If it seems that there is no risk of further damage to the youth and that families are able to engage in respectful dialogue about the youth's gender expression, separate sessions may not be necessary and family sessions may be appropriate from the beginning. **Table 1** provides clinical decisions made in the Steven and Julie/Dylan cases. Note that because of the significant conflicts within the family regarding Steven's gender identity and expression, separate sessions are recommended. The level of family attunement and support for Julie/Dylan's identity necessitates that therapy sessions include the entire family.

**Table 1**

**Applying stage one to the case examples**

| The Suarez Family | The Jackson Family |
|---|---|
| • Begin therapy with separate sessions because of the low level of attunement.<br>• Individual sessions with Steven are important initially because Steven has been exposed to extensive negative messages in his family system and needs a safe space until parents move toward affirming his experience of gender.<br>Sessions with parents:<br>• Parents begin to express their concerns in session with clinician.<br>• Explore parents' beliefs about gender and decipher what is harmful and what is affirmative.<br>• Parents explore role of religion, race, and ethnicity.<br>• Steven's mom processes feelings of guilt because she describes that before Steven was born she wished she would have a little girl. Stephen's father wonders if he was not a good enough male role model.<br>• Normalize parents' feelings, educate about the spectrum of gender expressions and identities, and normalize Steven's current expression of gender.<br>• Parents are encouraged to find safe spaces for Steven to explore and express his gender nonconformity.<br>• Parents express feelings of loss around the child they thought they had.<br>• Invite grandparents to session to help them understand Steven's gender expression and explore how they can become a resource for him.<br>• Role play ways of disclosing Steven's gender nonconformity with other family members and church community.<br>• Parents begin to move toward advocacy with increased confidence.<br>• Parents attend support group for parents of TGNC youth.<br>Sessions with Steven:<br>• Clinician enquires about Steven's preferred name and pronouns (Steven; he/him/his) and asks him to inform the clinician if it ever changes.<br>• Steven uses play to explore and express gender identities (eg, puppets, drawing, dress-up).<br>• Steven begins to express fears and challenges at school and home.<br>Conjoint sessions:<br>• Parents and grandparents continue work toward increased attunement, affirmation, and advocacy for Steven. | • Begin therapy with joint sessions including parents and child because parents were ultimately trying to support their child and not communicating harmful messages about gender.<br>• Enquire about chosen name and pronouns (Dylan; he/him/his). Clinician adopts new language immediately, explaining to parents the gender-affirmative approach.<br>• Parents and Dylan discuss fears about what lies ahead.<br>• Clinician provides education about the spectrum of gender expressions and identities.<br>• Invite Dylan's twin brother to join sessions; clinician provides education and a safe space for James to express any concerns and to learn new strategies for supporting Dylan in shared spaces.<br>• Dylan's twin brother joins a sibling group at a local LGBTQ center while parents attend a support group for parents.<br>Sessions with parents alone:<br>• Dylan's parents process feelings of disappointment and loss regarding the future of the daughter they thought they had.<br>• Parents express concerns and fears for the safety of their child and what the future of their child may look like.<br>• Clinician normalizes these feelings and emphasizes the protective impact their support will have for Dylan.<br>Sessions with Dylan:<br>• Dylan develops new coping strategies for self-harming behaviors and depressive symptoms.<br>• Clinician affirms Dylan's gender and externalizes the problem as transnegative societal messages. |

In some cases, the youth may not need treatment at all. When the child is not in any imminent risk, meaning there are no self-harming behaviors or other symptoms present, it may be more appropriate that the child does not attend therapy. Therefore, the child's life is minimally interrupted and the message is not sent that their gender is a problem. In such cases, treatment focuses on the family members who are struggling to accept and understand the gender expression. Other times, it may be important for the youth to have sessions alone to have a space in which their gender is affirmed and respected.

## Working with Parents

### Therapy as an isomorphic process

In most cases, the most important work to be done is with the parents and the clinician begins by making the therapeutic relationship with the parents a priority. The assumption is that an isomorphic process will take place; if the clinician can create a safe, accepting, supportive, and loving space for parents, then parents will be more apt to provide this for their child. This can sometimes be challenging for clinicians, because parents may be expressing views that contradict the clinician's views, such as gender nonconformity being pathologic. Clinicians should allow space for parents' views to be expressed, paying close attention to the love and concern that often underlies negative attitudes toward their child's gender expression. It is this love and concern that will act as building blocks for the rest of the therapeutic work.

Clinicians can assist parents of TGNC children and adolescents by reinforcing the notion that their primary role and responsibility as parents is to provide safety and support. Just as youth are in the therapy room to build resilience, so too are parents. An important task for therapists is to engage the parents in a process of creating immunity in the family against an outside world that at times is harsh and abusive toward TGNC persons. The clinician initiates this task by modeling a safe haven for the parents. Many families have felt blamed or shamed by others for their child's gender nonconformity. It is crucial to help parents understand that as a clinician, you assume that parents want what is best for their children. Sometimes what parents are doing with the intention of protecting their child, such as invalidating or prohibiting gender expression, is actually harming their child further. It is imperative to acknowledge that most children and adolescents do not have much agency to change difficult life situations. Parents are the main stakeholders in a child's life and they are the gatekeepers to the child attending therapy or getting medical treatment of any kind. A strong therapeutic relationship between the clinician and parents is most effective in helping the youth.

### Educating about the importance of family support

Parents exist in a context, in an era, in family, racial/ethnic, and religious or spiritual cultures that inform their view about what is "normal" and "valued" regarding gender identity and expression. They are informed by a society that has historically viewed gender nonconformity as a pathology. It may be difficult for parents to imagine their child on a path that may have tremendous challenges, including being misunderstood, discriminated against, and possibly being targets of violence. These prelearned beliefs and fears about TGNC people often get in the way of parents being able to support their child's gender journey.

Clinicians should educate parents about the current research on transgender people, which does indeed indicate that they often experience lower quality of life; increased suicide attempts; higher rates of depressive and anxious symptoms; family challenges; sexual and physical violence; poverty; and transgender-related discrimination in health care, housing, and employment.[6-12] However, research also suggests that parental support is a vital protective factor for children, buffering these harmful impacts of minority stress. Those who experience high parental rejection may be at increased risk for suicide ideation and attempts, depression, illegal drug use, alcohol abuse, smoking, homelessness, and engaging in unprotected sex and sex work, whereas those who experience parental support may experience higher self-esteem, social support, general health status, school belonging, academic achievement, life satisfaction, and overall mental health.[9,13-16] Making parents aware that their level of support may have a serious impact on their child's mental and physical health outcomes is another way of appealing to their desire to protect their child.

### Processing parents' emotions

It is common for parents to come to session wondering what they have done to cause their child's gender expression and may feel guilt for allowing or encouraging noncon-forming behaviors. They may also present with fear for their child's safety and feelings of disappointment, embarrassment, anxiety, confusion, anger, and concern.[1,17] It is important to maintain an affirmative approach and explain that their child's gender identity does not have a cause, rather their gender expression is a natural variation. Feelings of loss are often especially intense for parents of TGNC children. Some parents describe the grieving process as a necessity to let go of the fantasy they had for their child and to make room for the realities of the child they do have. Parents of TGNC commonly must mourn the loss of their hopes and dreams for their children and mourn the perceived loss of one child while another child emerges.[18]

The clinician's role is to help families feel heard, validated, and respected as they move through the series of complex emotions that often accompany raising a TGNC child. It is hoped this process will help them begin to move toward a more productive responsibility, which is to learn how to support their child. Once the clinician has helped them sit with their difficult feelings, the clinician can begin to help them expand their viewpoints.

### Expanding parents' views on gender

Fully engaging the parents in a conversation about how they developed their under-standing of gender and how it may have been informed by culture, race/ethnicity, religion, and class are key components to guiding the parents to a fuller understanding of gender. As parents explore the origins of their beliefs, the clinician can gently challenge them to see how their views may be hurtful to their child. The clinician simultaneously provides newer, accurate education about gender development, expression, sexual orientation, and other pertinent concepts.[3] The clinician helps parents understand that sharing hurtful beliefs with the child is extremely damaging to their sense of self-worth, and helps the family look for openings in their belief systems that provide useful building blocks to acceptance. In some families, parents' views on the TGNC child differ from each other and may be causing conflict in the couple or coparenting relationship. For example, one parent may be attuned with the child's gender expression, whereas the other parent opposes it. Therapy should address these differences with the goal of each parent expressing compassion for the other's views and together achieving increased attunement. In the case of Steven, some of the family's expectations about gender roles and norms were rooted in their Spanish/Uruguayan and Catholic back-grounds. Therapeutic discussions included how gender roles in these cultural contexts tend to be traditional, where masculinity and heterosexuality are absolute expectations of boys and men. Discussing the influence of these cultural beliefs allowed for the therapist to begin to expand these beliefs, encouraging parents to be more flexible.

It is common for families to feel isolated in the process of learning how to support their TGNC child and connecting them to resources can be relieving and educational. Clinicians should become acquainted with local resources that have gender-affirming programs, which may include support groups for the TGNC child, parents, and sometimes siblings. For example, PFLAG is an organization common to many communities, providing support to families of LGBTQ people. For some families, however, local educational and social resources may not be available and can instead be found online, such as Gender Spectrum (genderspectrum.org), a helpful resource for parents of TGNC youth. Additionally, clinicians can recommend various books.[18–20]

### Focusing on the journey, not the outcome

Parents often question the future outcome of their child's gender expression. They may wonder if their child will wish to transition socially or medically, whether a child is actually capable of making such a decision, and what may happen if their child experiences regret about this decision. They may worry about their child's safety and future relationships. Again, clinicians should remain compassionate and patient while the parents express their concerns and worries; this is an opportunity to help parents tolerate not knowing the end result.

The goal is to assist the family in responding to their child's gender journey in the moment with compassion, patience, and support. When parents' anxiety is decreased, they can have more control over their fears and can recognize that their needs are separate from their child's needs.[1] This ultimately makes space for parents to begin to listen to what their child is telling them about their experiences of gender. It is imperative that the parents feel heard by the clinician in the therapy room so this will take place. It is hoped that an isomorphic process will take place between the parents and clinician and then the parents and their child. In this case, the child should begin to feel heard, supported, and understood by their parents. It is recommended that the clinician continue to remind the parents along the way that the more they support their child and respond in loving and affirming ways, the more resilience their child will build.

### Working with Siblings and Other Family Members

Siblings must be carefully considered during the process of therapy. Sometimes, siblings experience less distress and confusion after being told about the gender identity/expression than parents, possibly because they are less invested than parents are in a sibling's outcome.[3] It is also typical that they have been exposed to more information regarding the complexities and possibilities of gender expression because of the generation in which they are growing up. However, siblings can struggle with feelings of loss, similar to that of parents, and clinicians can discuss, for example, what it feels like to lose a sister and also what it feels like to gain a brother. They may also struggle in the school setting if their sibling is being bullied and they want to protect them or they may be being bullied because of the sibling's gender expression. It is not uncommon for siblings to need some individual sessions in addition to participation in family sessions for support in these areas. Clinicians can help siblings figure out how to deal with this stress (eg, how to advocate for their sibling or how to diffuse situations). Importantly, the clinician and parents should help coach siblings to never contribute to the victimization of their TGNC sibling.

Some siblings might also be feeling like all of their parents' energy is being focused on how to cope with and what to do about the TGNC child's expression. This can leave siblings feeling like their needs are unimportant. For example, how can a daughter's quarrels with her best friend or a son's pressures to smoke cigarettes compare with a child that is dealing with gender transition? Furthermore, they may feel unackowledged for their accomplishments, much as success in school or in sports, because the family's attention is on the TGNC child. Clinicians can help parents understand that because one child is learning to navigate a gender journey, it does not mean siblings need less attention.

Although siblings are typically the most common family members (after parents) that need to be engaged in therapy to increase attunement, sometimes other family members may also be important to include. For example, grandparents often play a large role in families and may have a lot of influence over parents' beliefs about their child's gender expression. Any family member who is being affected by the child's gender should be invited to attend therapy, particularly if they are experiencing or creating distress in the family system. For example, in the case of Steven, the grandparents were identified as significant sources of support and thus became engaged in therapy to cultivate this support regarding Steven's gender expression.

### Working with Transgender and Gender-Nonconforming Children and Adolescents

Separate sessions for the child may be warranted if parents have not yet moved to a place of support and protection for their child. Another reason may be because the child has requested space of their own to explore or process their gender experience. It is also recommended that the child engage in individual therapy sessions in cases where the child is at-risk and is without family support. In therapy, the child or adolescent is encouraged to express their gender in any way that feels most comfortable for them. The clinician can inquire about what name and pronouns seem to fit best for them and the clinician adopts these preferences immediately. The clinician can also inform the child that therapy is a place to try new things, such as names, expressions, and pronouns. Many adolescents use therapy to express fears and to develop new strategies to deal with difficult situations or conversations. The goal is to move toward joint sessions when the child or adolescent and their parents are ready. Individual sessions may be a space to ready themselves for family sessions, practicing how they might express their feelings and needs to family members.

### Family Sessions

The goal of family sessions is for the family to incorporate the child's gender expression. Families are considered ready for joint sessions when the parents have done the therapeutic work required to respond to their child with love and support. Initial sessions may focus on repairing bonds, where parents really listen to their child. The child or adolescent will have also done significant therapeutic work to be able to articulate their experience to their parents. The clinician guides this interaction by helping the child or adolescent honestly express themselves and to help parents hold back any negative reactions. Once the family experiences healthy interactions, the parents and child can begin to move to stage two of therapy, where they can explore options for the child to experience increased comfort in their gender expression.

### STAGE TWO: EXPLORING AND SUPPORTING GENDER EXPRESSION/TRANSITION OPTIONS

The second stage of family therapy happens after there has been adequate time in which to assess and aid in the enhancement of family attunement. This stage involves exploring options for how the child can more congruently express their gender and, for some children, this may involve beginning a process of social and/or medical gender transition. Discussed next are strategies for working with youth when parents are not ready to affirm their gender, the role of distress and persistence in pursuing gender transition, the clinical readiness process to support gender transition, and guiding families in disclosing to others and advocating for the needs of their TGNC child.

### When Parents Are Not Ready to Affirm Gender Expression

When parents do not achieve adequate attunement, they may not be willing to consider options for gender expression or transition. Sometimes this is the case even after engaging in family therapy, when parents are strongly rooted in a gender binary belief system. This is especially difficult for younger children because they are often totally dependent on their parents to advocate for their gender expression/transition. Adolescents, however, often have other sources of support, such as friends and access to online resources. When it becomes clear that parents are not going to affirm their child's gender and that exploring options for gender expression and transition is not an option, clinicians can talk with the child about strategies for coping. Clinicians are an affirming voice in the child's life, assuring them that there is nothing wrong with them and that when they get older, they will be able to make their own decisions. Children without family support are at high risk for negative mental and physical health outcomes. Clinicians should develop a crisis plan with children, including who they can talk to or how they can self-soothe if they become self-harming/suicidal, with the intention of preventing or thwarting later self-harming/suicidal actions.

### The Role of Distress and Persistence in the Urgency of Gender Expression/Transition

When exploring options for gender expression/transition, TGNC youth express varying levels of urgency to begin social and medical gender transition. In gauging this urgency and how to move forward with families, it is important to keep in mind the role of distress and persistence. Distress refers to the discomfort and dysphoria being experienced by the youth. Although some youth are not distressed by their current body and gender expression, other youth may be so distressed that they are depressed; anxious; engaging in serious self-harming behaviors; or experiencing suicidal ideations, intents, or plans. Persistence refers to how diligent the youth is about their gender identity and the presence of a consistent history around this identity. **Table 2** provides a description of treatment with the Jackson family, where Dylan embodies this notion of persistence. He demonstrates consistency in his male gender identity, asks his parents to use a male name and pronouns, comes out as transgender at school, and expresses a desire for masculinizing hormone treatment.

If distress and persistence are present, other risks, such as youth changing their minds later, may be less important than the immediate reduction of the youth's distress. Adolescents in this category (as opposed to children) may require the most urgency to intervene medically, because their bodies are changing in ways that may cause permanent psychological damage and physical incongruence. When youth do not demonstrate persistence, they may still be distressed and it is important to assess whether the lack of persistence may be caused by depression or hopelessness. The gender transition process is demanding financially and emotionally. When depressive symptoms are present in TGNC children and adolescents this often disrupts motivation and goal-directed behaviors. In these cases, the depression should be treated and the readiness process (described later) should begin to explore the best options for the youth's happiness.

Sometimes distress is not present, but TGNC youth are persistent. These youth may be living in a gendered body and role that does not feel good, but they might not really recognize it because it's all that they know. They may know that they will feel better if they can transition, but also may express being able to "figure it out" if they cannot

| Table 2 Applying stage two to the case examples | |
|---|---|
| The Suarez Family | The Jackson Family |
| • Steven is not expressing that he feels that he is or wants to be a girl. Rather, he just wants to be able to express femininity. Thus, steps toward gender transition are not pursued.<br>• Clinician facilitates conversations about Steven's desires to wear feminine clothing and paint his nails sometimes.<br>• Coached by the clinician, parents express that it is okay that Steven express these feminine parts of self, but also talk about how he may be treated at school.<br>• At first, the family decides to experiment with feminine behaviors at home; mom bonds with Steven over doing his nails and shopping for girls' clothes.<br>• As the family becomes more comfortable, Steven begins to express himself outside of the home, wearing pink shoes and painted nails to school and to extended family gatherings.<br>• Clinician role plays with Steven and parents how to respond when comments about Steven's gender presentation are made.<br>• Steven seems visibly happier as he feels supported by his parents. | • Parents begin to use male pronouns and the chosen name Dylan.<br>• Dylan explores new ways of expressing gender identity and how to ask parents for what he needs.<br>• Role play difficult dialogues about gender and disclosure with family, friends, and peers.<br>• Dylan comes out as transgender at school and joins the school's LGBTQ group.<br>• Parents and Dylan attend meeting with school personnel; before attending, clinician discusses topics that are likely to come up in the meeting and seeks Dylan's input on what he would feel most comfortable with at school.<br>• Dylan expresses wanting to start masculinizing hormones and distress about looking younger than the other boys and hating his period and breasts.<br>• Parents discuss fears about hormones; clinician provides education about hormones.<br>• Family engages in readiness process to begin hormone therapy.<br>• Family discusses the possibility of chest reconstruction surgery in the future. |

transition. Clinicians should help youth navigate an identity that allows them the most access to joy, again beginning the readiness process. "Figuring it out" is not a state of joy. Adults later in life that have "figured it out" but have not lived happy lives often transition later, and therefore have a lot of loss to process about the life they did not live. When youth do not demonstrate distress or persistence, the strategy should be to wait and see what happens. Parents sometimes struggle in this stage because they have read or heard that gender transition will "fix" the problem for their child and they do not want their child to waste their life away in the wrong gender. These parents are well-meaning, wanting to support their child; however, gender transition should always be the choice of the person going through it. Some GNC youth do not ultimately desire gender transition and may express a gender outside of the gender binary or eventually become more comfortable with their assigned gender. **Fig. 1** illustrates the role of distress and persistence and how they impact decisions about gender transition.

### Readiness Process for Social and Medical Gender Transition

When considering gender transition, it is helpful to think about the process as being social and medical and that every path toward gender transition is unique. Some people decide to make social changes, such as adopting a chosen name and pronouns; some also make medical changes, such as hormone therapy; and some may choose to take only social or only medical steps in gender transition. In therapy, clinicians can

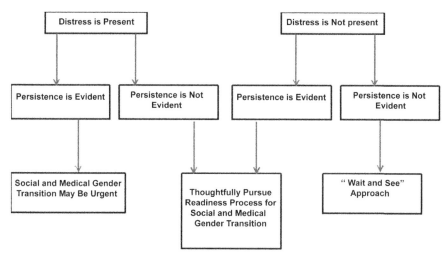

**Fig. 1.** Distress and persistence and their role in gender transition decisions.

explore with youth and families what steps, if any, make sense in order for the youth to feel more congruent in their expression. Often the first conversation with families is regarding a chosen name and pronouns. Some families are willing and able to immediately begin using the child's chosen name and pronouns in all settings. For some youth who are not out in all contexts, it may make the most sense to first begin using the name and pronouns only in the home. Other social changes that can be discussed are clothing, haircuts, chest binding for transgender young men, and shaving for transgender young women. Clinicians can facilitate conversations between family members, where children can verbalize their needs for certain gender expressions and parents can express any concerns they may have.

When families are considering medical gender transition for youth, it is often necessary for them to obtain a letter of support from a mental health professional as recommended by the Standards of Care (Version 7) of the World Professional Association of Transgender Health,[21] thus the clinician should formally engage in the readiness process for medical treatments. Prepubertal children may be experiencing distress in anticipation of the physical changes they will experience when puberty begins and therefore may want their puberty delayed medically. Adolescents may already be feeling discomfort and dysphoria because of their body changing and may wish to be begin hormone therapy that is congruent with their affirmed gender. Coolhart and coworkers[22] developed a clinical tool for youth and families to assess their client's readiness for transition. Domains to be explored include early awareness of gender and family context, parental/family attunement, current gender expression, school context, sexual/relationship development, current intimate relationships, support, and future plans/expectations. Consulting this resource is recommended for clinicians who are unfamiliar or inexperienced in this process.

## Disclosing to Others and Advocacy

Clinicians can also support families as they consider how to disclose the child's gender identity to extended family members; friends; teachers, administrators, and other school personnel; religious communities; and so forth. Role plays for difficult dialogues, new scenarios, and conflicts may be a helpful option to equip the family with the tools they may need to respond to others as they react to the child's gender. The child, boundaries around parental interventions, and when needed, the clinician can step in and assist with advocacy as appropriate. The school setting often presents the biggest challenges with regard to the child being able to use bathrooms and locker rooms that are comfortable and safe for them, and with school personnel and peers adopting the youth's chosen name and pronouns. For a thorough discussion of how clinicians can advocate in the school setting, see Coolhart and MacKnight.[23]

## SUMMARY

When families of TGNC youth seek therapy, engaging parents and often other family members in treatment is vitally important. Only when families can reach a level of attunement with the child's gender can the child truly thrive and feel protected from some of the mistreatment they may face in larger society. Clinicians have the opportunity to help families heal and grow, expanding their beliefs about gender, and helping their child explore gender expressions that are comfortable and congruent for them. Although this process is often challenging, it can result in families having more flexible and authentic relationships where all members feel valued for exactly who they are.

## REFERENCES

1. Malpas J. Between pink and blue: a multi-dimensional family approach to gender nonconforming children and their families. Fam Process 2011;50(4):453–70.
2. Hidalgo MA, Ehrensaft D, Tishelman AC, et al. The gender affirmative model: what we know and what we aim to learn. Hum Dev 2013;56:285–90.
3. Coolhart D. Helping families move from distress to attunement. In: Meier C, Ehrensaft D, editors. The gender affirmative model: a new approach to supporting gender non-conforming and transgender children. American Psychological Association; 2017.
4. Stone Fish L, Harvey RG. Nurturing queer youth: family therapy transformed. New York: W. W. Norton & Company; 2005.
5. Ehrensaft D. Gender born, gender made: raising healthy gender-nonconforming children. New York: The Experiment; 2011.
6. Bradford J, Reisner SL, Xavier J. Experiences of transgender-related discrimination and implications for health: results from the Virginia Transgender Health Initiative Study. Am J Public Health 2013;103(10):1820–9.
7. Budge SL, Adelson JL, Howard KA. Anxiety and depression in transgender individuals: the roles of transition status, loss, social support, and coping. J Consult Clin Psychol 2013;81(3):545–57.
8. Goldblum P, Testa RJ, Pflum S, et al. The relationship between gender-based victimization and suicide attempts in transgender people. Prof Psychol Res Pract 2012;43(5):468–75.
9. Grant JM, Motett LA, Tanis J, et al. Injustice at every turn: a report of the national transgender discrimination survey. Washington, DC: National Center for Transgender Equality and National Gay and Lesbian Task Force; 2011.
10. Kenagy GP. The health and social service needs of transgender people in Philadelphia. Int J Transgend 2005;8(2/3):49–56.
11. Newfield E, Hart S, Dibble S, et al. Female-to-male transgender quality of life. Qual Life Res 2006;15:1447–57.
12. Nuttbrock L, Hwahng S, Bockting W, et al. Psychiatric impact of gender-related abuse across the life course of male-to-female transgender persons. J Sex Res 2010;47(1):12–23.

13. Ryan CR, Huebner D, Diaz RM, et al. Family rejection as a predictor of negative health outcomes in white and Latino lesbian, gay, and bisexual young adults. Pediatrics 2009;123(1):346–52.
14. Ryan C, Russell ST, Huebner D, et al. Family acceptance in adolescence and the health of LGBT young adults. J Child Adolesc Psychiatr Nurs 2010;23(4):205–13.
15. Travers R, Bauer G, Pyne J, et al. Impacts of strong parental support for transgender youth. A report prepared for Children's Aid Society of Toronto and Delisle Youth Services. 2012.
16. Watson RJ, Barnett MA, Russell ST. Parental support matters for the educational success of sexual minorities. J GLBT Fam Stud 2016;12(2):188–202.
17. Lev AI. Transgender emergence: therapeutic guidelines for working with gender variant people and their families. Binghamton (NY): The Haworth Press, Inc; 2004.
18. Brill S, Pepper R. The transgender child: a handbook for families and professionals. San Francisco (CA): Cleis Press; 2008.
19. Ehrenhaft D. The gender creative child: pathways for nurturing and supporting children who live outside gender boxes. New York: The Experiment; 2016.
20. Testa RJ, Coolhart D, Peta J, et al. The gender quest workbook: a guide for teens and youngadults exploring gender identity. Oakland, CA: New Harbinger Publications; 2015.
21. Coleman E, Bockting W, Botzer M, et al. Standards of care for the health of transsexual, transgender, and gender-nonconforming people, version 7. Int J Transgend 2012;13(4):165–232.
22. Coolhart D, Baker A, Farmer S, et al. Therapy with transsexual youth and their families: a clinical tool for assessing youth's readiness for gender transition. J Marital Fam Ther 2013;39(2):223–43.
23. Coolhart D, MacKnight V. Working with transgender youth and their families: counselors and therapists as advocates for trans-affirmative school environments. Journal of Counselor Leadership and Advocacy 2015;2(1):51–64.

# Therapeutic Issues with Transgender Elders

Lynne Carroll, PhD, ABPP[a,b,*]

## KEYWORDS

- Transgender • Elders • Psychotherapy • Midlife transitioning • Elder services

## KEY POINTS

- Transgender (Trans) and gender nonconforming (TGNC) elders are an underrepresented group in contemporary research.
- TGNC-specific research is needed regarding the relationship between gender transition and age-related illnesses; polypharmacy and the potential for drug interactions; and sexual behavior, human immunodeficiency virus transmission patterns, and safer-sex programs for older TGNC adults.
- For TGNC persons the decision to transition is often postponed until retirement because of apprehension about job discrimination.
- Clinicians need to take on an advocacy role and become knowledgeable about health care providers and LGBT organizations and resources that are affirmative and be willing to advocate for TGNC elders.
- The shortage of geropsychologists and other health and social services personnel who are adequately trained to provide gender affirmative services for transgender elders poses considerable challenges for the future.

Despite the increased visibility of transgender and gender nonconforming persons (TGNC) in the United States, TGNC elders remain overlooked.[1,2] This circumstance is especially disconcerting given a significant increase both in the general elder population as well as an increase in numbers of TGNC persons who are electing to transition in their later years.[3] For many gender nonconforming older adults the decision to transition in later life is driven by societal changes in attitudes, particularly among younger cisgender persons, as well as other factors, such as phase of life.[4,5]

To a large extent the challenges and rewards associated with aging are universal regardless of gender identity and sexual orientation. Irrespective of culture, the experiences of cognitive and physical limitations, challenges of caregiving both in families of origin and of choice, loss of friends and social networks, and end-of-life issues,

Disclosure Statement: The author has no conflict of interest and is not receiving any funding.
[a] University of North Florida, Department of Psychology, 1 UNF Drive, Jacksonville, FL 32244, USA; [b] Independent Practice, 13111 Atlantic Boulevard, Suite 2, Jacksonville, FL 32225, USA
* University of North Florida, Department of Psychology, 1 UNF Drive, Jacksonville, FL 32244.
E-mail address: lcarroll1258@gmail.com

Psychiatr Clin N Am 40 (2017) 127–140
http://dx.doi.org/10.1016/j.psc.2016.10.004
0193-953X/17/© 2016 Elsevier Inc. All rights reserved.

confront most adults as they age. However, as the evidence presented in this article demonstrates, the multiple effects of stigmas surrounding age, gender identity, and sexual orientation significantly impacts the aging experience, both positively and negatively.

To a large extent aging services providers, including those in long-term care facilities and in-home services, assume that elders are heterosexual and fit neatly into the gender binary. The fears that are common among lesbian, gay, and bisexual (LGB) adults about aging, such as living in isolation, being neglected or abused by health care providers, and harassed by their cisgender peers, are even more acute in TGNC elders, especially among those whose trans identities are more detectable.[6] The purpose of this article is to provide mental health clinicians with practical input about psychotherapeutic issues for use with TGNC elders. A summary of current research findings as well as an overview of historical and contemporary trends in the clinical treatment of TGNC clients is provided. A case vignette is presented that draws on the author's clinical experience as a lesbian-identified psychologist who works with older adults and more specifically with TGNC elders. This vignette illustrates the ways in which sociocultural and historical contexts impact a trans woman's decisions about transitioning in later life. Lastly, recommendations are also provided for mental health practitioners, many of whom are likely to encounter TGNC elders.

## A SNAPSHOT OF TRANSGENDER OLDER ADULTS

The challenges associated with constructing a snapshot of transgender elders in the United States are significant. Estimates of the current TGNC population aged 65 years and older range anywhere from 700,000[3] to 2.8 million.[7] It is predicted that by 2030, one in 5 Americans are projected to be aged 65 years and older and that the number of TGNC elders will steadily increase.[8]

Christine Jorgensen was one of the first trans women in the United States to undertake gender-confirming surgery (GCS) in the 1950s. Although she achieved some degree of celebrity status during her lifetime, most TGNC persons to follow were forced to hide their gender identities in order to avoid discrimination. The prevailing aim of treatment among clinicians in the 40+ years following Jorgensen's groundbreaking surgery was to help trans persons reject their pretransition identities and erase their histories.[9] Consequently, an unknown portion of TGNC older adults blended into the mainstream society, hiding their identities to maintain jobs or families.[3,10] Historically, this process connoted the completion of medical procedures to enable a female or male gender expression. At present, TGNC persons are beginning to expand the consciousness of the rest of the population of what it means to transition.

Gender transition or the gender-affirmation process has come to be understood more broadly as "an interpersonal, interactive process whereby a person receives social recognition and support for their gender identity and expression."[11] GCS may or may not be part of a person's transition process, and some TGNC persons may make few if any physical changes and live outside the binary. A growing consciousness exists, especially among younger cohorts, that a range of gender identities between and outside of the categories of male and female exists. Yet, despite these shifts, it is important to note that TGNC elders belong to an aging culture that adheres to binary constructions of gender.[12]

## RESEARCH CHALLENGES

Transgender elders are one of the most underrepresented groups in contemporary research.[4] Finkenauer and colleagues[13] conducted a comprehensive review of the published research between 1992 and 2012, using a total of 15 databases. Only 20% of these articles incorporated samples of participants who were TGNC older adults aged 50 years or older.[13] Up until quite recently, the scant research on TGNC elders has been obtained from convenience samples that were overrepresented with educated white persons living in urban areas. The lack of visibility of trans participants in the research is, in part, exacerbated by several problematic methodological practices, including combining samples of sexual and gender minority elders under one umbrella obscuring possible differences between subgroups.[13] Researchers had conflated data from trans samples and thereby ignored potential variation in experiences of trans women and trans men. The practice of collapsing the different groups of trans persons older than 50 years into one category labeled *old* has obscured possible variations between age groups. As a result of this practice very little is known about TGNC persons older than 85 years. There is also a dearth of research that specifically addresses the aging experiences of TGNC elders who have conservative religious affiliations or live in rural communities.

Historically, research has focused singularly on transgender identity obscuring the fact that TGNC persons experience multiple forms of oppression at the same time based on race, ethnicity, age, class, disability status, and sexual orientation.[14] This practice contributed to the invisibility of TGNC persons of color. de Vries,[15] for example, noted that scholars have too often attended to "what (White) trans people's experiences can tell us about (White) cisgender experience, often at trans people of color's expense."[15] The growing focus on intersectionality theory in social science research has created opportunities for scholars to describe the ways in which oppressive institutions (ie, racism, sexism, transphobia, ageism, classism, and so forth) intersect. According to intersectionality theory these stigmas cannot be examined separately or ranked in terms of their degree of oppression.[16] For example, elder trans women of color likely face transphobia, racism, sexism, and ageism.

Lastly, far too little attention has been paid to the important relationship between aging and gender transition and such age-related illnesses as heart disease, diabetes, and osteoporosis. We know little about the difficulties associated with hormone replacement therapy (HRT) and aging.[13,17] The issues surrounding polypharmacy and the potential for dangerous drug interactions in older adults who have undergone HRT and are currently receiving treatment of age-related illnesses require further understanding.[18,19] There is also a lack of knowledge specific to heightened human immunodeficiency virus/AIDS risks among trans older adults and a lack of research specifically on sexual behavior, transmission patterns, and safer-sex programs.[13,20]

## COMPARATIVE RESEARCH FINDINGS: TRANSGENDER AND GENDER NONCONFORMING AND LESBIAN, GAY, AND BISEXUAL ELDERS

In 2011, the combined efforts of the National Gay and Lesbian Task Force and the National Center for Transgender Equality resulted in the largest study of transgender persons in US history referred to as "Injustice at Every Turn."[21] Of 6400 participants, 11% were aged 55 years and older. Most of those respondents had been living in their affirmed gender for just a few years. Of trans elders 65 years of age and older, 70% reported having delayed gender transitioning to avoid discrimination in employment.[21] As many as 8% of participants 65 years and older versus 20% of participants' aged 55 to 64 years reported that they had been refused care by a health care provider because of their gender identity.[21] Approximately 11% of elders older than 65 years and 12% of participants between 55 and 64 years of age reported having experienced verbal harassment or disrespect in a physician's office or hospital.[21] This mistreatment was magnified among respondents with lower income levels and respondents who were people of color. Latino respondents reported the highest rate of unequal care among any racial/ethnic category with 32% citing unequal care from a doctor or hospital and 19% in emergency departments or mental health clinics, whereas African American transgender respondents were among the most vulnerable to physical assault in hospitals and doctors' offices.[21]

The first national, federally funded study entitled Caring and Aging with Pride: The National Health, Aging and Sexuality Study was undertaken to address quality of life for 2546 LGBT adults aged 50 years and older.[22] This study revealed that LGBT older adults have higher rates of mental health issues and disabilities than their cisgender counterparts.[22] When TGNC older adults are compared with LGB elders, TGNC older adult participants had significantly poorer health in terms of overall physical health, disability, depressive symptoms, and perceived stress. They also reported significantly lower incomes,[22] greater risk for unemployment and poverty, and higher rates of discrimination and victimization[21] and had less access to health care and health insurance than their LGB counterparts.[23]

Trans elders must confront multiple and cumulative impacts of a range of negative responses, including emotional repulsion, microaggressions, discrimination, and violence. Cook-Daniels[24] posited that transgender elders face risks that LGB elders do not typically experience in terms of the possibility of being placed in residential care, using medical and assistive services, such as bathing and dressing, which require them to disrobe and out themselves. The fear of rejection and discrimination deters TGNC from seeking such needed assistance. Transgender persons, regardless of age, often do not have a regular physician and must, therefore, rely on emergency room and urgent care physicians for immediate health care needs. Many transgender persons live with untreated or undertreated chronic conditions, such as hypertension or diabetes. Furthermore, fear of revealing their transgender identity may prevent adequate health screenings, such as for breast or prostate cancers. Treatable health conditions may increase in severity unnecessarily because of the reluctance of transgender people, young and old, to confront prejudice in the health care system.[23] This circumstance may be particularly true for transgender elders who were among generational cohorts that were raised to passively accept the authority of medical professionals.[23] Younger generations generally seek medical care armed with medical information from the Internet and a more questioning attitude toward physician's directives for care.[25]

## THE EVOLUTION OF THERAPY WITH TRANSGENDER AND GENDER NONCONFORMING PERSONS: FROM OPPRESSIVE TO AFFIRMATIVE

Current estimates indicate that 75% of TGNC persons of all ages use psychotherapy,[21] a rate 25 times that of their cisgender counterparts.[26] Despite these numbers, clinically oriented graduate programs provide only minimal training necessary not only to work with older adults[27] but most especially with TGNC persons.[28] There is a lack of evidence-based therapy approaches and resources specifically for use with transgender older adults, with the exception of recent articles detailing cognitive behavioral approaches.[29] Elder care personnel receive minimal if any training and have limited familiarity with the needs of TGNC elders. It is no wonder that trans elders remain closeted when they receive community-based elder services, such as long-term care and home care.[30] Given the lack of adequate training as well as the projected noticeable shortage of geriatric health and social services personnel not only for the general population of elders but also more specifically for transgender elders, considerable challenges await the helping professions in the future.[31]

Mental health services for transgender persons, regardless of age, have historically focused on diagnosis and treatment of psychopathology. Much of the literature focused on the Standards of Care (SOC) developed by the World Professional Association for Transgender Health.[32] Initially, these standards were applied to those who met the diagnostic criteria for gender identity disorder.[33] Transgender persons approached mental health practitioners with the intent of gaining access to treatments, such as GCS, breast removal, breast augmentation, hormone therapy, electrolysis, and facial feminization. Therapists protected their clients from undergoing medical treatment unprepared and protected physicians from litigation in the event that their clients were not prepared for the results of surgery or other medical procedures.[34] As a result, therapy was not viewed as a place to address life challenges and instead served as an access point to medical intervention. It is important to underscore that such practices excluded transgender people who did not undergo medical procedures from mental health treatment altogether.[34]

As a result of a lengthy history of being pathologized and disempowered by the psychiatric profession, subject to humiliating treatment or having treatment withheld, it is likely that many TGNC elders may have a deep distrust of mental health professionals.[34] Mental health professionals have been positioned as gatekeepers to medical treatment of TGNC persons because the transitioning process required a psychological assessment, diagnosis, and a letter confirming that these interventions are medically and psychologically necessary. Historically, TGNC persons resented the requirement to be seen by a mental health professional in order to have access to medical treatment. This history is particularly problematic when TGNC older adults come to therapy now after having had negative interactions with therapists in the past.[35] In many cases it may require more time to form a strong, positive psychotherapeutic alliance with TGNC elders.

As the SOC have become more flexible in version 7,[32] clinical practice has shifted from a primary focus on diagnosis and transition to more inclusive quality-of-life issues, such as lifelong preventive and primary care. The diagnosis of gender identity disorder has been supplanted in the *Diagnostic and Statistical Manual of Mental Disorders*, Fifth Edition by that of gender dysphoria.[36] The latter is used when one experiences significant distress due to disparity between gender identity and sex assigned at birth. Access to transition-related care and being able to transition (legally, socially, and/or medically) is indeed life saving for many TGNC individuals.

Significant changes in the standards for clinical practice provide opportunities for a more affirming approach to treatment and transition. As preceding review demonstrates, most TGNC elders came of age in times whereby past discrimination and marginalization were the norm and now face a phase of life that often necessitates great reliance on health and social service agencies. Therefore, mental health clinicians must be specially equipped to act as advocates for their TGNC elders by facilitating access to appropriate care and resources with compassion and sensitivity.[35]

## EMBRACING A TRANS AFFIRMATIVE PERSPECTIVE IN PRACTICE, RESEARCH AND ADVOCACY

Although Terri's story is similar to and overlaps those of other TGNC elders, there are a myriad of clinical issues that were not addressed in this case vignette. For example, specific challenges for mental health professionals include working with TGNC elders who have chronic age-related illnesses, those with dementia and other cognitive

*The following case study outlines the progression of outpatient psychotherapy over the span of 1 year with a 58-year-old trans woman assigned male at birth who is of mixed European heritage. Terri (a pseudonym) is the principal caregiver for her biological mother, who is in her 80s. Both reside in a politically, religiously, and socially conservative region in the Southeastern United States. Terri identifies as bisexual. Terri was married and divorced while in her 20s. Terri identifies herself as a woman only in the safety of the therapy room. Terri disclosed that she occasionally wears women's makeup and clothing only in the privacy of her bedroom. Following Terri's retirement from the armed forces, she was employed in a manufacturing job for several years. Terri has a history of substance abuse and subsequent treatment. She has continued to maintain her sobriety without relapse for several years. Terri is the eldest of several siblings. Her biological parents were divorced in her childhood, and she has been her mother's sole source of economic and social support for the past several years. Terri's mother has significant chronic health problems.*

*Terri initially presented with symptoms consistent with a diagnosis of recurrent major depressive disorder. Terri reported that she previously sought therapy for her depression but discontinued treatment after only a few sessions because she felt apprehensive about disclosing her gender identity to her therapist. Terri's feelings of anxiety and distrust are not uncommon among elder trans persons who have endured lifetimes of discrimination.*

*During our first session, I provided Terri with a brief professional biography, which included my professional and community service activities in LGBT organizations. Special care was taken to provide a safe and nonjudgmental climate and to use appropriate pronouns throughout our sessions together. Contemporary psychodynamic theory was used to guide Terri's treatment. According to Lin Fraser,[37] this approach is especially useful with TGNC clients given the fact that so often gender identity, a core component of selfhood, is negated and hidden from others and a false self develops in its place. Many transgender persons develop a false sense that is hypermasculine or hyperfeminine. According to Fraser, "the person develops that self in secret and alone and, to avoid stigma, often hides this again after coming out."[37] This secrecy and the lack of witnessing and mirroring often required for healthy ego development to occur, frequently leads to mistrust of feelings, depression, social withdrawal, and substance abuse. Acceptance of one's transgender identity may be "the end point of a long internal struggle to preserve secrecy."[37] Like many TGNC elders, Terri was aware very early in her life of the incongruence between her body and her internal sense of gender. Terri had the sense of herself as female but learned through experience to suppress this. Terri recalled her strong desire and delight in dressing up like a girl. She recalled that one of her siblings accidently discovered her while crossdressing in her childhood and told on her. Throughout her school years, Terri continued to feel uncomfortable with her body and gender assigned at birth. The chronic name-calling and bullying that ensued left psychic scars, much like those described in prior research with TGNC interviewees when they crossed gender norms and were subject to gender policing by the larger society.[4]*

*As a young adult Terri joined the military in an attempt to fulfill expectations of her gender assigned at birth. Interestingly, research demonstrates that significant numbers of TGNC persons have histories of military service.[38–40] Among male-to female (MTF) individuals, the attraction toward the military is especially keen because of the emphasis on traditional masculine values. Terri, like many other MTFs, was striving to embody societal ideals of traditional masculinity.[39,40] Contrastingly, for female-to-male individuals, the military offers a setting where taking on more traditionally masculine roles is viewed as acceptable behavior.[41] Terri recalled serving in the military and having to cope with repeated demeaning antigay harassment from fellow soldiers who assumed that she was a gay man. These experiences triggered deep shame and compounded the self-loathing she felt in her childhood. Terri coped with these feelings by abusing substances. In this respect, Terri's story mirrors those of many other TGNC persons whose first experiences of rejection and discrimination are associated with homophobia. For example, in their qualitative study of 45 TGNC adults by Mizock and Hopwood,[42] interviewees recalled multiple experiences of homophobic transphobia, defined as "the stigmatization of transgender individuals based on the confounding of sexual orientation and gender identity."[42]*

Per evidence-based research and recommendations of clinicians,[43,44] I incorporated Meyer's[45] minority stress model in therapy to helping TGNC adults like Terri to understand why so many TGNC persons experience mental health issues. This model posits that gender nonconformity is not itself pathologic but it is the actual exposure to chronic stressors, such as social and employment discrimination, that results in depression, anxiety, and other disorders. Concomitantly, it is the anticipation and vigilance required to ward off such possibilities as well as the internalization of negative feelings about oneself as TGNC that promotes further stress.

Terri, like many TGNC persons who serve in the military, are potentially exposed to combat-related trauma as well as transphobic related discrimination and violence. They are especially at risk for trauma-related conditions, such as posttraumatic stress disorder.[46] Trauma scholars have written extensively about trauma in a way that is informative to clinicians who treat sexual and gender minorities. Traumatic events are categorized as intrapersonal (self-inflicted violence), interpersonal (occurring between 2 or more people), and collective (violence inflicted by institutions).[47] Researchers have also acknowledged that repetitive exposure to oppression associated with transphobia, referred to as insidious trauma, can lead to the development of symptoms associated mood disorders and substance abuse.[47] Terri's experiences of trauma were cumulative and reverberated throughout the developmental stages of her life. Like other survivors of trauma, Terri benefited from learning stress-reduction techniques (eg, diaphragmatic breathing, progressive muscle relaxation), becoming more comfortable identifying emotional states, learning how to identify and effectively express emotions, regulating emotions, and tolerating distress.[48]

Terri's depression was sometimes immobilizing for her. Terri reported gender dysphoria and experienced significant discomfort with her body. Because of her recurrent depression and history of substance abuse, it was necessary to conduct ongoing assessments for suicidal risk and relapse. Terri was able to identify that underlying her depression were feelings of frustration and anger at herself for, in her words, "taking so long to transition." She expressed deep regret about not having transitioned earlier in her life. It was important to reframe this self-blaming stance by reminding Terri of her resiliency in the face of past trans discrimination and noting considerable sociocultural shifts in attitudes and advancements in gender-affirming treatment.

In our sessions Terri dealt actively with universal and existential issues, which are consistent with many older adults at her phase of life. Terri's anxiety related to her own mortality and concerns about having squandered valuable time were important catalysts for her decision to seek therapy. Her decision to disclose her gender identity in therapy was also based on a sense that she was now entering a phase of her life in which she would be better emotionally and financially equipped to begin her gender-affirmation process. Terri had worked extensively with the local Veteran's Administration in order that they might fund the tuition regarded to obtain her bachelor's degree. Terri also thought that the local university would be a safer place in which to transition rather than risking discrimination on the job.

Terri's fears about discrimination are echoed in the research cited earlier. As result of postponing transition until later in life, many TGNC have been able to maintain careers without being discriminated against.[21] This sentiment is also reflected in the narratives of Siverskog's[4] research participants, some of whom chose the time after retirement to transition partly because they "perceived this as a time where one is able to choose the social context in which one wants to be in."[4] For many TGNC elders the decision to transition is driven by both individual and societal changes. Fabbre[5] also posits that among older transgender adults, existential awareness of death is a contributing factor in the timing of the decision to transition in midlife.[5] One of the significant variables reported by participants in Fabbre's study was the awareness of "limited days in which to embrace one's authentic self" and to feel "congruent within oneself, and face death with a sense of having truly lived."[5]

In addition to the recognition that her risks of employment discrimination were diminished after retirement, it is also important to note that Terri's desire to transition was determined by other sociocultural factors. Because of recent advances in the Veteran's Health Administration policies regarding gender-affirmative medical care, hormone therapy, and preoperative evaluations, Terri had a greater sense of optimism about financial affordability and accessibility of these services.[40] It is important to note that not all TGNC veterans are afforded this possibility, as there is state-by-state variability in these services.[49]

Throughout therapy, Terri expressed anxiety and dread about coming out as both transgender and bisexual to her mother. Terri's commitment to caregiving for her elderly and frail mother was a significant factor in deciding not to come out to her mother and in her postponement of HRT. Terri's willingness to sacrifice her own needs in order to protect her mother is consistent with prior research findings. For example, Simon and colleagues[50] explored both transgender and cisgender participants' recollections of parenting behaviors and maladaptive core beliefs. Transgender participants represented themselves as more isolated and more focused on the needs of others than their cisgender counterparts. Simon and colleagues[50] attributed these findings to the observation that many trans persons feel forced to suppress their core sense of themselves for fear of rejection. As the eldest child in her family of origin, Terri's self-sacrifice was very strong. Terri disclosed her belief that she needed to compensate for the many financial and emotional disappointments her mother had experienced throughout her lifetime. Terri thought that no sacrifice was too great in the service of caring for her mother. Terri specifically expressed the fear that the possible emotional strain dealing with her transition would likely compromise her mother's health status. Ironically, during Terri's therapy, her mother experienced a minor health crisis and shortly thereafter, Terri experienced health problems of her own, which were potentially brought on by stress. When Terri recovered and returned to therapy she realized that this experience was a reminder that she was not going to be an effective caretaker for her mother if she did not care for herself. Despite the rather obvious cognitive dissonance, Terri did not disclose to her mother her gender identity.

Terri's ambivalence about her telling her mother continued to be a major theme in therapy. We discussed how Terri might better prepare and set the stage for this disclosure. To this aim, Rosenfeld and Emerson's[51] process model was presented to Terri because it provided a framework for understanding the grieving process that parents and family members often experience when transgender loved ones come out. Transgender persons, regardless of age, can appreciate the ways in which their own process of discovery and self-acceptance is parallel and mirrored in the Kübler-Ross'[52] (1969) bereavement stages of denial, anger, bargaining, depression, and acceptance.[51,52] Teri was asked in therapy to stage the conversation with her mother. Terri was given a homework assignment to compose an unsent letter to her mother in which she comes out to her mother regarding both aspects of her identity as a woman and as bisexual. During the following session Terri arrived bearing a copy of her letter, which reportedly took her several hours to complete. This experience was emotionally cathartic and enabled Terri to work at her own pace while also facilitating her empowerment and emotional processing.

Terri, like many TGNC persons, had done extensive research on the Internet locating trans-affirming information and social networking sites. These resources serve as lifelines for TGNC persons. Like many trans persons, Terri accessed important information about the gender transition process from the Internet. Before initiating therapy, Terri had explored her gender identity without benefit of personal contact and engagement with another trans-identified person, which is somewhat common given Terri's age and the relatively conservative nature of the geographic region in which she lives. For example, in Beemyn and Rankin's[53] large-scale study of TGNC persons, 25% of their sample aged 50 years and older knew another transgender person when they self-identified as such. This finding is in contrast to 75% of participants 18 to 22 years of age who met another transgender person.[53] I provided Terri with the contact information of a local transgender activist who was willing to serve as a mentor to other TGNC persons. Information about LGBT community events was also provided, including a particular event in which a transgender activist was a principal guest speaker.

Terri was initially excited about these opportunities but often cited reasons why she would not attend and/or after the fact she offered excuses for missing these events. After several weeks in therapy, Terri was encouraged to attend a newly formed community support group for TGNC persons, which met monthly. Terri postponed attending the group for several months each time offering an excuse for why she could not attend. It was clear that she was not ready, and it took several months before she attended her first meeting. This attendance was considered a therapeutic breakthrough because the trans community was one of the only sources of belonging and connectedness available to Terri.[54]

Sanchez and Vilain[55] studied the impact of collective self-esteem as a coping mechanism for transgender individuals experiencing psychological distress. They found that the more positively TGNC persons felt about their community, the less psychological distress participants experienced. TGNC-specific support groups and social networks that promote connectedness to this community can serve as a counterpoint to the microaggressions and discrimination often experienced.[43] Research substantiates that transgender persons who have prior contact with other trans persons are significantly less anxious, evidence less suicidality, and are more comforted than those who have had no prior contact.[56]

It is important to note, however, that in addition to internal struggles about coming out, older TGNC persons are often isolated from identification and involvement with gay and lesbian communities. As has been reflected in the research, LGBT organizations and activities tend to be youth oriented.[57] Intergenerational connections are challenging when LGBT youths have negative attitudes toward elders, and elders have difficulty relating to younger persons who have had very different experiences with and attitudes regarding LGBT identity and disclosure.[58,59] For example, young gay men in one study defined old as 39 and above.[60]

It is important to emphasize that Terri's gender-affirmation process is ongoing. As of this date, Terri has still not initiated hormone therapy despite giving her trans-affirmative health care referrals and she has not talked to her mother. Terri's readiness for or ambivalence about change was sometimes expressed by canceling her therapy appointments. Fraser[37] warns that therapy with TGNC clients can take a long time with the therapist acting as a mirror for the TGNC client. Terri's case illustrates the importance of therapists assessing and monitoring countertransference issues. In their discussion of clinical issues, Rachlin and Lev[61] address a similar therapeutic dynamic associated with TGNC clients who chose to remain closeted. They note the tension between some in the trans community that would view the choice to stay in the closet as inauthentic. Similarly, I sometimes felt frustrated in working with Terri and aware of the potential of placing undue pressure on her to transition. I sometimes thought that Terri's decision to protect her mother by living as a man was problematic because, for so many TGNC persons, starting or completing the transition process eased their distress, depression, and suicidal ideation and behavior. Despite my personal feelings of impatience, I also felt compelled to respect the self-disclosure strategies she used to preserve her relationship with her mom and to ensure her sense of safety. I was also forced to examine ways in which my own privileges and experiences contributed to my countertransference reactions. Although I have at times felt marginalized as a lesbian, my privilege as a white, traditionally gendered or cisgender, currently able-bodied person who was raised with economic privilege contributed to my feelings of impatience.

Terri's case provides awareness around the reality that not all older TGNC persons are disenfranchised from their families of origin. Regardless of their experience in disclosing to families, many TGNC older adults serve important caregiving functions to family members.[62,63] Prior research findings report that a rather large percentage of LGBT adults serve in caregiving capacities both within their families of origin and choice. For example, in the Metlife Mature Market Institute and the Lesbian and Gay Aging Issues Network of the American Society of Aging[64] survey of more than 1200 lesbian and gay (LG) adults, LG elders are twice as likely to serve as a caregiver for a parent, family member, partner, friend, or neighbor and to spend significantly more hours per week providing that care, when compared with their heterosexual counterparts.[56]

Terri's story not only depicts the challenges of transitioning in later life but also illustrates the potential advantages of doing so. Terri possessed a strength and resilience that is prominent among many LGBT persons who are able to age more successfully than their heterosexual and cisgender counterparts because of having learned to successfully manage stigmatized identities. A lifetime of managing stigma and coping with the stresses of marginalization may inure LGBT individuals to the difficulties faced by many heterosexuals and cisgender persons as they age.[6] Kimmel's[6] term "crisis competence" is aptly used to these cases whereby the process of managing stigmatized identities earlier in life can lead to the enhanced ability of TGNC elders to adapt and to thrive during old age.[6]

limitations, and those who are facing end-of-life decisions.[7,49] Practitioners will need to be sensitive to the needs of TGNC elders whose cognitive abilities diminish their capacities to provide informed consent to treatments, such as HRT and GCSs.[7,49]

The issues that TGNC elders face are complex. The requirements of gender affirmative practice necessitate that clinicians validate the full spectrum of gender identities and expressions and consider the impact of multiple identity statuses, such as race, ethnicity, class, and disability status, at different life stages and historical contexts.[65,66] In essence, clinicians must be better able to address countertransference issues as they arise and accommodate the heterogeneity of TGNC elders. It is imperative that mental health professionals identify physicians and other health care providers who are trans affirmative and be equipped to work within interdisciplinary professionals, such as geriatric care physicians, endocrinologists, and other health care specialists. Consultation, collaboration, and case management are important skill sets necessary for work with TGNC elders. Practitioners need to be knowledgeable about LGBT organizations and resources that specifically target TGNC elders and most especially TGNC elders of color. Given the significant financial challenges that many TGNC elders experience, it is imperative that practitioners keep abreast of insurance and Medicare-related changes and inform their clients of these.[49]

As has been previously noted, research is needed to inform practice. At present, there is a lack of evidence-based therapy approaches and specifically for use with transgender older adults. Research is needed to further elucidate the important relationship between aging-related illnesses, such as heart disease, osteoporosis, and HRT.

Terri's case illustrates the necessity for clinicians who work with TGNC older adults to move beyond the therapy room and into the larger community. As practitioners we are required to advocate for trans rights and promote awareness regarding issues that transgender elders face.[67] This shift in perspective is radical because it means developing skill sets often not taught in clinically oriented graduate programs. Community psychologist Isaac Prilleltensky[68] has been particularly outspoken about the need for psychology and human services professionals to strike a balance between individual and collective wellness by eliminating oppressive social and political conditions.[68] Porter and colleagues[49] stressed the need for mental health practitioners to address the institutional barriers, such as the lack of policies related to housing TGNC elders who reside in long-term care facilities. Advocating for and helping aging transgender persons to advocate for their rights to be treated with dignity and respect is critical for those working with TGNC elders. Clinicians can play integral roles by advocating for state and local legislation that prohibits discrimination based on gender identity and expression that will benefit the growing population of aging TGNC adults. Policies that prohibit expressions of homophobia, biphobia, and transphobia and training that reinforce those policies particularly as they affect TGNC elders will be needed.

Elder care agencies will be challenged to deliver services in contexts where ageism, transphobia, homophobia, and biphobia render sexual and gender minority elders invisible and alienated from their two natural allies: LGB and mainstream senior communities. Ironically, those most likely to possess negative attitudes toward TGNC elders in senior centers and residential and other long-term care facilities are cisgender peers. All elder service providers and clinicians must provide safe and welcoming environments for TGNC elders that accommodate their desired gender, in part, through the provision of education to cisgender coresidents. It is also advisable whenever possible for TGNC persons to be included in visible roles as facilitators of transpositive educative programs and trainings.

## REFERENCES

1. Benson KE. Seeking support: transgender client experiences with mental health services. J Fem Fam Ther 2013;25:17–40.

2. Persson DI. Unique challenges of transgender aging: implications from the literature. J Gerontol Soc Work 2009;52(6):633–46.

3. Witten TM, Eyler AE. Transgender and aging: beings and becomings. In: Witten TM, Eyler AE, editors. Gay, lesbian, bisexual and transgender aging: challenges in research, practice and policy. Baltimore (MD): Johns Hopkins University; 2012. p. 187–269.

4. Siverskog A. "They just don't have a clue": transgender aging and implications for social work. J Gerontol Soc Work 2014;57(2–4):386–406.

5. Fabbre VD. Gender transitions in later life: the significance of time in queer aging. J Gerontol Soc Work 2014;57(2–4):161–75.

6. Kimmel D. Lesbian, gay, bisexual, and transgender aging concerns. Clin Gerontol 2014;37(1):40–63.

7. Witten TM. When my past returns: loss of self and personhood – dementia and the trans person. In: Westwood S, Price E, editors. Lesbian, gay, bisexual and trans individuals living with dementia: theoretical, practical and rights-based perspectives. New York: Routlege Press; 2015. p. 110–23.

8. Orel NA, Fruhauf C. The intersection of culture, family, and individual aspects: a guiding model for LGBT older adults. In: Orel NA, Fruhauf C, editors. The lives of LGBT older adults. Washington, DC: American Psychological Association; 2015. p. 3–24.

9. Katz-Wise S, Budge SL. Cognitive and interpersonal identity processes related to mid-life transitioning in transgender women. Couns Psychol Q 2013;28(2):150–74.

10. Cook-Daniels L. Transaging. In: Kimmel D, Rose T, David S, editors. Lesbian, gay, bisexual and transgender ageing: research and clinical perspectives. New York: Columbia University Press; 2006. p. 290–335.

11. Sevelius JM. Gender affirmation: a framework for conceptualizing risk behavior among transgender women of color. Sex Roles 2013;68(11–12):675–89.

12. Witten TM. Graceful exits: intersection of aging, transgender identities, and family/community. J GLBT Fam Stud 2009;5:35–61.

13. Finkenauer S, Sherratt J, Marlow J, et al. When injustice gets old: a systematic review of trans aging. J Gay Lesbian Soc Serv 2012;24(4):311–30.

14. Parent MC, DeBlaere C, Moradi B. Approaches to research on intersectionality: perspectives on gender, LGBT, and racial/ethnic identities. Sex Roles 2013;68:639–45.

15. de Vries KM. Transgender people of color at the center: conceptualizing a new intersectional model. Ethnicities 2015;15(1):3–27.

16. Nadal KL, Davidoff KC, Davis LS. A qualitative approach to intersectional microaggressions: understanding influences of race, ethnicity, gender, sexuality, and religion. Qual Psychol 2015;2(2):147–63.

17. Ferron P, Young S, Boulanger C, et al. Integrated care of an aging HIV-infected male-to-female transgender patient. J Assoc Nurses AIDS Care 2010;21(3):278–82.

18. Berreth ME. Nursing care of transgendered older adults: implications from the literature. J Gerontol Nurs 2003;29(7):44–9.

19. Blank TO, Asencio M, Descares L, et al. Aging, health, and GLBTQ family and community life. J GLBT Fam Stud 2009;5(1–2):9–34.

20. Cook-Daniels L, Munson M. Sexual violence, elder abuse, and sexuality of transgender adults, age 50+: results of three surveys. J GLBT Fam Stud 2010;6(2):142–77.

21. Grant JM, Mottet LA, Tanis J, et al. Injustice at every turn: national trans discrim ination survey. Washington, DC: National Center for Trans Equality ad National Gay and Lesbian Task Force; 2011.
22. Fredriksen-Goldsen KI, Cook Daniels L, Kim HJ, et al. Physical and mental health of transgender older adults: an at-risk and underserved population. Gerontologist 2013;54(3):488–500.
23. Cahill S, South K, Spade J. Outing age: public policy issues affecting gay, lesbian, bisexual and transgender elders. New York: National Gay and Lesbian Task Force Policy Institute; 2000.
24. Cook-Daniels L. Transgender aging: what practitioners should know. In: Orel NA, Fruhauf CA, editors. The lives of LGBT older adults. Washington, DC: American Psychological Association; 2015. p. 193–216.
25. Berkowitz EN, Schewe CD. Generational cohorts hold the key to understanding patients and health care providers: coming-of-age experiences influence health care behaviors for a lifetime. Health Mark Q 2011;28(2):190–204.
26. Budge SL. Interpersonal psychotherapy with transgender clients. Psychotherapy 2013;50(3):356–9.
27. Hinrichsen GA, Zeiss AM, Karel MJ, et al. Competency-based geropsychology training in doctoral internships and postdoctoral fellowships. Train Educ Prof Psychol 2010;4:91–8.
28. Singh AA, Boyd CJ, Whitman JS. Counseling competency with transgender and intersex clients. In: Comish JA, Schreier LA, Nadkami LH, et al, editors. Handbook of multicultural competencies. Hoboken (NJ): Wiley & Sons, Inc; 2010. p. 415–42.
29. Austin A, Craig SL. Transgender affirmative cognitive behavioral therapy: clinical considerations and applications. Prof Psychol Res Pr 2015;46:21–9.
30. Fruhauf CA, Orel NA. Conclusion: fostering resilience in LGBT aging individuals and families. In: Orel NA, Fruhauf CA, editors. In the lives of LGBT older adults. Washington, DC: American Psychological Association; 2015. p. 217–27.
31. Stanley IH, Duong J. Mental health service use among lesbian, gay, and bisexual older adults. Psychiatr Serv 2015;66(7):743–9.
32. Coleman E, Bockting W, Botzer M, et al. Standards of care for the health of transsexual, transgender, and gender-nonconforming people, version 7. Int J Transgend 2012;13(4):165–232.
33. American Psychiatric Association (APA). Diagnostic and statistical manual of mental disorders, text revision (DSM-IV-TR). 4th edition. Washington, DC: American Psychiatric Association; 2000.
34. Lev AI. Transgender emergence: therapeutic guidelines for working with gender variant people and their families. Binghamton (NY): Haworth Clinical Practice Press; 2004.
35. Moody C, Peláez S, Fuks N, et al. "Without this, I would for sure already be dead": a qualitative inquiry regarding suicide protective factors among trans adults. Psychol Sex Orientat Gend Divers 2015;2(3):266–80.
36. American Psychiatric Association. Diagnostic and statistical manual of mental disorders: DSM-5. 5th edition. Arlington (VA): American Psychiatric Publishing, Inc; 2013.
37. Fraser L. Depth psychotherapy with transgender people. Sex Relation Ther 2009; 24(2):126–42.
38. Brown GR. Transsexuals in the military: flight into hypermasculinity. Arch Sex Behav 1988;17(6):527–37.
39. Johnson L, Shipherd J, Walton HM. The psychologist's role in transgender-specific care with U.S. veterans. Psychol Serv 2015;13(1):69–76.

40. McDuffie E, Brown GR. 70 U.S. veterans with gender identity disturbances: a descriptive study. Int J Transgend 2010;12(1):21–30.
41. Lehavot K, Simpson TL, Shipherd JC. Factors associated with suicidality among a national sample of transgender veterans. Suicide Life Threat Behav 2016;46(5):507–24.
42. Mizock L, Hopwood R. Conflation and interdependence in the intersection of gender and sexuality among transgender individuals. Psychol Sex Orientat Gend Divers 2016;3(1):93–103.
43. Maguen S, Shipherd JC, Harris HN, et al. Prevalence and predictors of disclosure of transgender identity. Int J Sex Health 2007;19(1):3–13.
44. Hendricks ML, Testa RJ. A conceptual framework for clinical work with transgender and gender nonconforming clients: an adaption of the minority stress model. Prof Psychol Res Pr 2012;43(5):460–7.
45. Meyer IH. Prejudice, social stress, and mental health in lesbian, gay, and bisexual populations: conceptual issues and research evidence. Psychol Bull 2003;129:674–97.
46. Burnes TR, Dexter MM, Richmond K, et al. The experiences of transgender survivors of trauma who undergo social and medical transition. Traumatology 2016;22(1):75–84.
47. Richmond KA, Burnes T, Carroll K. Lost in translation: interpreting systems of trauma for transgender clients. Traumatology 2012;18(1):45–57.
48. Linehan MM. Cognitive-behavioral treatment of borderline personality disorder. New York: Guilford Press; 1993.
49. Porter KE, Brennan-Ing M, Chang SC. Providing competent and affirming services for transgender and gender nonconforming older adults. Clin Gerontol 2016. [Epub ahead of print].
50. Simon L, Zsolt U, Fogd D, et al. Dysfunctional core beliefs, perceived parenting behavior and psychopathology in gender identity disorder: a comparison of male-to-female, female-to-male transsexual and nontranssexual control subjects. J Behav Ther Exp Psychiatry 2011;42(1):38–45.
51. Rosenfeld C, Emerson S. A process model of supportive therapy for families of transgender individuals. In: Denny D, editor. Current concepts in transgender identity. New York: Garland Press; 1998. p. 391–400.
52. Kübler-Ross E. On death and dying. New York: The Macmillan Company; 1969.
53. Beemyn G, Rankin S. The lives of transgender people. New York: Columbia University Press; 2011.
54. Barr SM, Budge SL, Adelson JL. Transgender community belongingness as a mediator between strength of transgender identity and well-being. Psychol Sex Orientat Gend Divers 2016;63(1):87–97.
55. Sanchez FJ, Vilain E. Collective self-esteem as a coping resource for male-to-female transsexuals. J Couns Psychol 2009;56(1):202–9.
56. Testa RJ, Jimenez CL, Rankin S. Risk and resilience during transgender identity development: the effects of awareness and engagement with other transgender people on affect. J Gay Lesbian Ment Health 2014;18(1):31–46.
57. Brotman S, Ryan B, Collins S. Coming out to care: caregivers of gay and lesbian seniors in Canada. Gerontologist 2007;47(4):490–503.
58. Barker JC, Herdt G, de Vries B. Social support in the lives of lesbians and gay men at midlife and later. Sex Res Social Policy 2006;3(2):1–23.
59. Hostetler AJ. Community involvement, perceived control, and attitudes toward aging among lesbians and gay men. Int J Aging Hum Dev 2012;75(2):141–67.

60. Schope RD. Who's afraid of growing old? Gay and lesbian perceptions of aging. J Gerontol Soc Work 2005;45(4):23–39.
61. Rachlin K, Lev AI. Challenging cases for experienced therapists. J Gay Lesbian Ment Health 2011;15(2):180–99.
62. Cronin A, Ward R, Pugh S, et al. Categories and their consequences: understanding and supporting the caring relationships of older lesbian, gay and bisexual people. Int SocWork 2011;54(3):421–35.
63. Gabrielson ML. 'We have to create family': aging support issues and needs among older lesbians. J Gay Lesbian Soc Serv 2011;23(3):322–34.
64. MetLife Study. Still out, still aging: the MetLife study of lesbian, gay, bisexual, and transgender baby boomers. 2010. Available at: https://www.metlife.com/assets/cao/mmi/publications/studies/2010/mmi-still-out-still-aging.pdf. Accessed July 15, 2013.
65. Carroll L, Gilroy PJ. Transgender issues in counselor preparation. Counselor Education & Supervision 2002;41(3):233–42.
66. Carroll L, Gilroy PJ, Ryan J. Counseling transgendered, transsexual and gender-variant clients. J Couns Dev 2002;80:131–7.
67. Carroll L. Counseling sexual and gender minorities. Upper Saddle River (NJ): Pearson; 2010.
68. Prilleltensky I. Value-based praxis in community psychology: moving toward social justice and social action. Am J Community Psychol 2001;29(5):747–78.

# Affirmative Cognitive Behavior Therapy with Transgender and Gender Nonconforming Adults

Ashley Austin, PhD, LCSW[a],*, Shelley L. Craig, PhD, LCSW[b],
Edward J. Alessi, PhD, LCSW[c]

## KEYWORDS

- Transgender • Gender nonconforming • Cognitive behavior therapy • Affirmative
- Minority stress

## KEY POINTS

- Transgender and gender nonconforming (TGNC) individuals continue to be a highly marginalized population, subject to transphobia that manifests in the form of stigma, discrimination, and victimization.
- An affirming and trauma-informed perspective recognizes that traumatic events and experiences, including non–life-threatening forms of transphobic prejudice, may threaten TGNC clients' sense of safety, power, and control over their lives.
- Trans-affirmative clinical practice acknowledges and counters the oppressive contexts of the lives of transgender individuals.
- Transgender-affirmative cognitive behavior therapy (TA-CBT) is a version of cognitive behavior therapy (CBT) that has been adapted to ensure (1) an affirming stance toward gender diversity, (2) recognition and awareness of transgender-specific sources of stress, and (3) the delivery of CBT content within an affirming and trauma-informed framework.

Transgender and gender nonconforming (TGNC) identities are gaining visibility in contemporary society. Although many of the more nuanced experiences of identifying as transgender remain obscured, there is growing recognition among researchers, clinicians, trans activists, and their allies that gender is multidimensional and not binary.[1,2]

Disclosure: The authors do not have relationships with any commercial companies that have a direct financial interest in the subject matter or materials discussed in this article or with a company making competing products.

[a] School of Social Work, Barry University, 11300 Northeast 2nd Avenue, Miami Shores, FL 33161, USA; [b] Factor Inwentash Faculty of Social Work, University of Toronto, 246 Bloor Street West, Toronto, Ontario M5S 1A1, Canada; [c] School of Social Work, Rutgers, The State University of New Jersey, 360 Martin Luther King Jr. Boulevard, Hill Hall, Room 401, Newark, NJ 07102, USA
* Corresponding author.
E-mail address: aaustin@barry.edu

In particular, although it is apparent that the opportunity to medically transition is a critical component of health and well-being for some transgender youth and adults, it is becoming clearer that there are multiple ways for TGNC people to live authentically. An increasing number of TGNC youth and adults are not interested in medically transitioning, feeling comfortable with a nonbinary presentation of their genders without the use of hormones or other medical interventions.[2] However, because TGNC identities and experiences continue to be marginalized, navigating a TGNC identity continues to be a complex process.[3] As a result of systematic discrimination, marginalization, and multiple forms of victimization, authentically expressing and navigating a TGNC identity can be a confusing and, at times, arduous and painful process. Persistent physical, emotional, interpersonal, contextual, financial, and other barriers can also complicate the path to living authentically.[3,4] Thus, psychiatrists, psychologists, social workers, and other mental health professionals play a key role in facilitating self-awareness, authenticity, and self-acceptance among TGNC individuals.[5] Therefore, this article introduces mental health clinicians to transgender-affirmative cognitive behavior therapy (TA-CBT). TA-CBT is a version of CBT that has been adapted to ensure practitioners recognize specific sources of stress among TGNC individuals and also to deliver CBT content within an affirming and trauma-informed framework.[6,7]

## MINORITY STRESS

In order to fully support TGNC clients in mental health settings clinicians must have a well-developed understanding of minority stress and its negative outcomes among TGNC clients. Although Meyer[8] initially applied minority stress theory to sexual minority populations, in recent years it has also been used to explain negative mental health outcomes among TGNC individuals.[9–11] The minority stress model is based on the notion that sexual and gender minorities encounter high levels of stress because of homophobic and transphobic social conditions. In turn, excess exposure to stress causes higher prevalence of psychological distress among sexual and gender minority individuals compared with cisgender/heterosexual individuals.[11]

TGNC individuals experience high levels of minority stressors, including verbal, physical, and sexual abuse; stigma; and internalized stigma.[4,12,13] Discrimination rooted in transphobia and cisgender privilege begins early, with TGNC individuals reporting alarming rates of verbal abuse and physical and sexual victimization.[4,14] Although schools provide the context for a lot of bullying and exclusion of TGNC youth,[15] victimization is not limited to "any particular social context as it pervades their school, family, religious, and community environments" (p. 228).[16]

## MENTAL HEALTH CONSEQUENCES

High levels of identity-based stigma and stress contribute to disparate mental health outcomes among the TGNC community.[9] TGNC individuals experience disproportionate rates of psychological distress, such as suicidality, depression, and anxiety, compared with their cisgender counterparts.[17–20] Growing research highlights particularly high rates of suicidality among TGNC individuals.[4,12,20,21] Nuttbrock and colleagues[20] found that 54% of participants had experienced suicidal ideation and 28% had previously attempted suicide. Even higher rates of attempted suicide (45%) were found among respondents (aged 18–24 years) in the National Transgender Discrimination Survey.[22] Furthermore, emerging research suggests that lifetime prevalence rates of nonsuicidal self-injury are also notably high (42%) among transgender adults in the United States.[18] The incidence of depression and anxiety is also increased among TGNC individuals.[17,19,20]

## TRAUMA AND POSTTRAUMATIC STRESS DISORDER

The marginalization of transgender identities increases their vulnerability to stressful events, including those of a life-threatening nature.[23] Understanding the effects of posttraumatic stress disorder (PTSD) and other trauma-related disorders is critical for providing culturally informed mental health care to TGNC individuals.[24] Although there have been few empirical studies of PTSD in transgender samples, preliminary evidence indicates that transgender persons who have been exposed to violence and other traumatic events experience high levels of posttraumatic symptoms.[23] Moreover, gender nonconformity in childhood is associated with greater exposure to potentially traumatic events and the subsequent development of PTSD.[25,26] Controversy persists in that many TGNC individuals show symptoms consistent with a PTSD diagnosis, but they are exposed to events that do not meet the definition of trauma in the *Diagnostic and Statistical Manual of Mental Disorders*.[24] Scholars have discussed the importance of recognizing the potential effects of so-called non-traumatic events, especially those involving prejudice, among sexual and gender minority populations.[27] Frequent exposure to non–life-threatening forms of transphobic discrimination in acute (eg, being fired from employment because of gender identity) or chronic forms (eg, dealing with transphobic stigma, and macroaggressions) can be accompanied by a pervasive fear of victimization.[24] This hypervigilance may in turn become a fundamental aspect of the person's transgender identity.[24] Empirical studies are still needed to investigate associations between PTSD and non–life-threatening forms of transphobia, but, given the high exposure to prejudice events among the transgender community, it is likely that this would be the case.[24]

Alessi and colleagues[27] discussed how current knowledge about the relation between nontraumatic events and PTSD among sexual minority individuals is informed by attempts to understand the psychological effects of prejudice events among people of color[28] and women.[29] For example, when persons of color encounter racial prejudice, regardless of whether these events involve actual or threatened death, they experience cognitive and affective assaults on identity that permeate their core sense of themselves.[28] There is mounting recognition that transphobic stigma, discrimination, and victimization may have a similar traumatic impacts on transgender individuals.[30,31] Advances in knowledge and understanding regarding the detrimental cognitive, emotional, physical, and neurobiological effects of traumatic experiences[32–34] underscore the importance of integrating a trauma-informed perspective when working with TGNC clients. An affirming and trauma-informed perspective recognizes that traumatic events and experiences, including non–life-threatening forms of transphobic prejudice, threaten TGNC clients' sense of safety and undermine self-determination. This perspective also seeks to restore TGNC clients' sense of personal safety, power, and control.

## FACTORS AFFECTING RESILIENCE

Despite the challenges that many TGNC individuals experience while navigating their stigmatized identities, factors such as transgender-affirmative social support, social connectedness, and self-advocacy can facilitate their resilience. Identity-affirming social support may contribute to healthy coping mechanisms[17,35,36] and protect against poor mental health (eg, anxiety and depression).[37] A sense of social connectedness with the broader transgender community contributes to increased comfort with a person's transgender identity and better behavioral health.[38,39] Social connectedness with the transgender community may be facilitated through the use of information and communication technologies (ICTs).[40] ICTs (eg, transgender-specific YouTube channels or Facebook groups) are frequently used to obtain transgender-specific knowledge (eg, understand transgender identities or locate trans-affirming doctors) and to connect with other transgender individuals,[41,42] when it is unsafe to be "out" in their physical environments.[40,43] In addition, self-advocacy such as educating others about transgender issues, advocating for transgender inclusion, and participating in transgender community–building activities can facilitate resilience.[44] Taken together, fostering resilience by enhancing trans-specific social support, social connectedness, and self-advocacy represents an important component of affirmative interventions for TGNC individuals.

## TRANSGENDER-AFFIRMATIVE CLINICAL APPROACHES

Affirmative approaches to clinical practice for TGNC individuals have emerged in response to unethical clinical practices intended to change, pathologize, or invalidate transgender identities and experiences.[6] The potential harm associated with reparative or conversion therapy is well documented,[45] particularly for TGNC youth,[46] and should be clearly rejected as a clinical option. In contrast, affirmative interventions, which support and validate the identities, strengths, and experiences of TGNC individuals, can promote health and well-being.[47] It is critical that clinicians adopt, and make known, an affirming clinical position that recognizes all experiences of gender as equally healthy and valuable.[6] Affirmative practice must acknowledge and counter the oppressive contexts of the lives of TGNC individuals.[27,48,49] Clinicians should attend to policies regarding access to services based on gender identity versus assigned sex at birth and the use of gender-neutral restrooms, the development of transgender-inclusive promotional materials (eg, pamphlets, Web pages), and the use of inclusive language on intake and other forms of documentation.

It is recommended that clinicians show gender inclusivity at the moment of first contact with their clients. For example, "Hello, my name is Beth and I use she, her, and hers pronouns; what is your name and preferred gender pronouns?" Unconditional positive regard for the diversity of transgender identities and expressions that is integrated throughout all interactions with transgender individuals is perhaps the most fundamental component of a transgender-affirmative (TA) clinical practice. As such, clinicians must diligently engage in self-exploration regarding their personal gender-related attitudes, beliefs, and biases. In addition, interventions attending to the specific needs of transgender individuals should be implemented and practiced with competency, and this requires clinicians who are committed to developing transgender-specific knowledge and skills. Transgender-affirmative cognitive behavior therapy (TA-CBT) and clinical considerations associated with competent implementation are discussed later.

## TRANSGENDER-AFFIRMATIVE COGNITIVE BEHAVIOR THERAPY

Cognitive behavior therapies (CBTs) have received extensive empirical support for use in the treatment of a variety of mental health issues with both adolescents and adults in multiple settings.[50,51] CBT has been successful in addressing depression, anxiety, substance abuse, trauma, and suicidality,[50,52–54] issues that disproportionately affect the transgender community. The underlying premise of CBT is that cognitions affect emotional and behavioral health. CBT is based on Beck's[55] seminal research on the relationship between maladaptive or unhelpful cognitions and depressive symptoms. CBT interventions are designed to improve emotional and behavioral functioning by targeting underlying problematic cognitions.[56]

TA-CBT is a version of CBT that has been adapted to ensure:

1. An affirming stance toward gender diversity
2. Recognition and awareness of transgender-specific sources of stress (eg, transphobia, gender dysphoria, systematic oppression)
3. The delivery of CBT content within an affirming and trauma-informed framework[6,7]

Given the traumatic experiences often precipitated by minority stress among TGNC individuals, a critical component of TA-CBT is that it is grounded in an understanding of the pervasiveness and consequences of transgender stigma and prejudice. In the presence of notable structural oppression, TA-CBT is designed to promote positive change and healthy coping through the creation of a safe, affirming, and collaborative therapeutic relationship. TA-CBT recognizes that, as result of pervasive exposure to transphobic attitudes, beliefs, and behaviors, transgender individuals may develop patterns of negative thinking about themselves.[9,57] The internalization of negative or stigmatizing thoughts then affects emotional and behavioral responses.

Clinicians who foster a trans-affirming view of transgender identities and experiences can help their clients overcome negative self-perceptions and views of the future. From a CBT perspective, embracing a trans-affirming worldview can decrease troubling emotional responses (eg, shame, anxiety) and subsequent maladaptive behavioral responses. One of the many benefits of TA-CBT is its flexibility, allowing an assessment of an individual's risk as well as resilience.[6,48,58] Components of TA-CBT, assessment and case conceptualization, self-regulation, psychoeducation, modifying thinking, and behavioral activation are discussed later.

### Components of Transgender-affirmative Cognitive Behavior Therapy

### Assessment and case conceptualization

An important component of CBT is understanding the clients' presenting issues within the context of early learning experiences, because these lead to the development of core beliefs that may contribute to and/or exacerbate current problems.[57] During the early phases of assessment and case conceptualization in TA-CBT it is important to explore clients' early experiences of recognizing and understanding their own gender identity. Because there is a general lack of tolerance for gender nonconformity or gender ambiguity in Western society, which historically has been exacerbated by the pathologization of transgender experiences by medical, mental health, and social service professionals,[59] children and adults are often shamed for being transgender or gender nonconforming and quickly learn to suppress and/or reject a transgender identity.[3] These early experiences can be traumatic and contribute to core beliefs of being unlovable, worthless, or incompetent. Core beliefs are conceptualized as a set of deeply embedded ideas that are regarded as absolute truths.[57] The core beliefs of TGNC clients are likely reinforced by negative social messages that marginalize and pathologize gender nonconformity.

A sensitive and in-depth exploration of these early experiences may be critical for people to understand current thoughts and beliefs about themselves and their identities (**Table 1**). This sort of exploration is helpful for uncovering early traumatic experiences associated with navigating an emerging transgender identity, as well as the ways in which the internalization of transphobic thoughts and beliefs contributed to a person developing these negative core beliefs. During assessment and case conceptualization, clinicians should explore clients' thoughts and beliefs about their transgender identities and experiences through sensitive and affirming questions. **Table 1** provides examples of such questions.

| Table 1 | |
| --- | --- |
| Trans-affirmative case conceptualization process | |
| Recommended Areas for Exploration | Suggested Questions |
| Explore early memories of recognizing and experiencing a TGNC identity | What was it like for you to recognize and understand your gender identity? What were some of your early messages about what it means to be a boy? A girl? Neither? What were some of your early messages from family/peers/school/media/religious leaders about TGNC people and identities? |
| Explore thoughts and beliefs about TGNC identity | How have you made sense of the early messages you received about being TGNC? How have you reconciled what your religion/family believed about being TGNC with your own beliefs? |
| Explore TGNC-specific stressors associated with transitioning | What are some of your concerns about coming out and/or transitioning? What are the components of transitioning that are causing you the greatest stress? What are some of the unexpected stressors associated with life posttransition? |
| Explore TGNC-specific stressors associated with being nonbinary in presentation and/or identity | What are some of your concerns about presenting as nonbinary in your daily life? What are some of the unexpected challenges and/or barriers to living authentically? |
| Explore TGNC-specific discrimination across life domains | Have you been experiencing any identity-specific discrimination or harassment at work, school, or in your community? Can you tell me what that has been like for you? Can you share any specific experiences of discrimination or harassment you face as a nonbinary person navigating your environment? |

When exploring stressors that may exacerbate client's presenting issues, it is important to explore transgender-specific stressors across multiple domains of life (eg, family, school/work, sexuality, spiritual life), as well as during the various phases of transitioning/living authentically (eg, pretransition, transition, or posttransition). In such instances, it may be useful for clinicians to explore stressors associated with the specific phase (see **Table 1**). Because nonbinary transgender clients may not conceptualize their experiences of living authentically through the lens of transitioning, it is important to remember that not all gender-diverse clients want to transition or seek services related to transitioning (see **Table 1**). These persons are often subject to more intense prejudice and discrimination. The words of one trans activist eloquently convey the continued and exacerbated oppression of nonbinary individuals in contemporary society: "What has become evident is that so many of us who do not pass as male or female are still regarded as disposable by both cis and trans communities."[60] It is important that TA clinicians have the competence to explore transgender-specific stressors in a way that invites discussion of the diverse range of transgender experiences.

### Self-regulation

The deleterious impact of traumatic experiences on the central nervous system and subsequent self-regulation is well documented.[34] Moreover, it is increasingly recognized that clients' inability to explore, process, and recover from traumatic experiences is facilitated by the ability to regulate their responses to stress.[34,61] The exploration of past and current stressors within the clinical setting may trigger intense emotional reactions for some clients whose experiences of transphobia in the home, school, and/or community were particularly traumatic. Thus, it is important that clinicians help clients achieve a relaxed body and mind before they begin to recount traumatic experiences. Strategies for teaching clients to self-regulate may include deep breathing, progressive muscle relaxation, or mindfulness.[62] Only when clients achieve a relaxed body and mind can they safely explore potentially traumatic histories that may be contributing to presenting clinical issues.[34,61]

### Psychoeducation

Once the clinician and the client have developed a shared understanding of the client's presenting concerns and the ways in which external stressors affect current issues, introducing TA psychoeducation is an important component of the TA-CBT process. There are 2 primary goals of the psychoeducational component in TA-CBT:

1. To help clients develop a basic understanding of the theoretic underpinnings of cognitive behavioral approaches to promoting health and well-being through an introduction to the cognitive model; that is, the relationship between thoughts, emotions, and behaviors
2. To help clients to understand the potentially traumatic impact of transphobic discrimination and prejudice and its contribution to feelings of distress

The psychoeducational component within TA-CBT provides the opportunity for clients to identify and explore painful and traumatic effects of discrimination, victimization, and violence within a supportive and safe environment. As clinicians begin to validate the difficult experiences of TGNC clients, clients may begin to interpret these experiences and resultant emotional or behavioral consequences through a trauma-informed, minority stress lens. In this way, clients can begin to move away from a view of themselves as abnormal, weak, or disordered toward a more accurate view of themselves as ordinary individuals navigating exceptionally stressful and often traumatic circumstances. It is also through this process that TA clinicians can focus on client resilience and the ways in which clients have been able to survive and adapt to severe minority stress.

### Modifying negative thinking

The CBT model posits that an individual's cognitive reactions to life experiences affect their emotions and behaviors. These cognitive reactions are often referred to as automatic thoughts, which are described as words, phrases, or images that spontaneously occur in an individual's mind in response to specific situations and circumstances.[57] CBT interventions are based on the premise that automatic thoughts are influenced by underlying core beliefs, as well as intermediate beliefs. Intermediate beliefs are defined as conditional rules, attitudes, and assumptions, often unspoken, that significantly affect the way in which individuals respond to life's challenges and stressors.[57] A critical component of most CBT interventions is to identify and modify automatic thoughts, as well as related intermediate and core beliefs, through the use of a variety of effective strategies.[57,63] One strategy that may be particularly important for transgender individuals is to evaluate the intermediate and core beliefs underlying their negative automatic thoughts within a transgender-affirming context. Negative core beliefs generally have one of the following 3 themes: being worthless, being unlovable, or being helpless or incompetent.[57] Beginning in childhood, TGNC individuals are exposed to many implicit and explicit messages that stigmatize and pathologize gender nonconformity and transgender identities. In many instances these messages are internalized, which can lead to the development of core beliefs of being worthless or unlovable (eg, "Being transgender is not valued, therefore I have no value"). These core beliefs yield intermediate beliefs in people that may include a rigid if/then style of thinking about themselves and their interactions with the world (eg, "If I am not perfect, no one will like me").

Intermediate and core beliefs are typically not accessible to clients at the start of therapy.[63] Therefore, the therapeutic work during this phase of treatment may include helping the client to recognize underlying intermediate and core beliefs through an exploration of some of the client's common automatic thoughts through the downward arrow method. **Fig. 1** shows this technique. The clinical data gathered during the TA case conceptualization phase of treatment (eg, early messages about gender identity) can be used to inform the client and clinician about some of the messages that may have led to core beliefs. For example, clients develop core beliefs of being

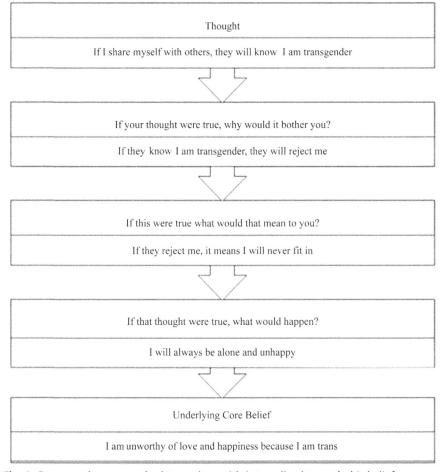

Fig. 1. Downward arrow method to explore with internalized transphobic beliefs.

worthless or unlovable after repeated early exposure to stigmatizing messages like "Stop being a sissy!"; "What's wrong with you?"; and "Look at that he/she."

In addition to exploring the genesis of these beliefs, clinical work might focus on exploring the ways in which clients' environmental contexts contribute to the maintenance of these negative beliefs. For example, many TGNC persons are members of faith communities and places of worship that are not affirming or welcoming. Many live in rural areas where there is little access to transgender resources and supports. In order to competently and effectively examine the reasons for the development and maintenance of negative core beliefs, it is necessary that clinicians have a comprehensive understanding of the minority stressors that promote and inhibit well-being among TGNC individuals.

Several general CBT techniques, including Socratic questioning and behavioral experiments, are also well suited for use with TGNC clients. These techniques can be used to decrease the intensity of negative core beliefs (eg, "I am worthless") and to increase the new core beliefs (eg, "I am worthy of love and life"; "I am resilient").[57] For example, a clinician may ask a client who holds the core belief "I am worthless" to write down specific pieces of evidence that support this statement (eg, "There is no place for nonbinary people in this world"; "I will never be a 'real' woman"; "Being trans has made me a disappointment to everyone in my life"), as well as pieces of evidence that counter this unhelpful core belief (eg, "At the gender equality center my perspective is valued and solicited because it is unique"; "My partner thinks I am beautiful exactly the way I am"; "My best friend and my sister are incredibly proud of my strength and courage"). Because negative messages about transgender people and identities are so pervasive, articulating and exploring counterevidence for the first time can be challenging but enlightening, decreasing, even slightly, the power of the negative core belief.

Another key component of this process is to help clients reframe the evidence that supports the core belief in order to diminish its impact. For example, a clinician might engage in cognitive restructuring with the client around what it means to be a "real" woman. The clinician and client may explore womanhood in a broad and inclusive context, challenging the notion that people must be cisgender to be a "real" woman and/or question whether there is such a thing as "real" woman. If the negative self-beliefs are deeply entrenched and the client is experiencing a great deal of distress, TA clinicians may need take an even more active role in treatment by explicitly challenging transphobia and cisgender privilege.

An additional approach to helping clients develop more affirming core beliefs is to validate transgender-specific stressors and foster their resilience.[48,64] To do so in an affirming manner, certain practices should be avoided when clients disclose incidents of discrimination.[48] For instance, clinicians must not automatically universalize experiences of discrimination (eg, "Not everyone is going to like us") or search for alternative reasons for the perpetrator's behavior (eg, "Perhaps he is just that way to everyone"). Such reactions may discount the reality and severity of transphobic discrimination in the lives of TGNC clients. In addition, clinicians must be careful not to minimize the feelings of pain, shame, or fear brought about as a result of transgender discrimination (eg, "Adversity will make you stronger"). This sort of response may be perceived as disrespectful or flippant, and misses the opportunity to explore emotional reactions to discrimination and marginalization that may be important to understanding the clients' clinical concerns. Particularly when clinicians are cisgender, such responses may be experienced as a subtle form of transphobia that has the potential to undermine the therapeutic relationship. Instead, when clients disclose incidents of transgender-specific stigma, discrimination, and oppression, they should ha addressed in a supportive and validating manner. Table 2 offers specific recommendations regarding clinical responses to use, as well as to avoid, when exploring transgender discrimination within the therapeutic context.

### Behavioral activation

Behavioral activation recognizes that environmental and contextual factors are often key sources of client issues and therefore directly targets client behaviors that are critical to alleviating distress and promoting well-being.[65] The goal of behavioral activation is to help clients engage in specific activities when they feel like they cannot (eg, go out and take a walk even when feeling unmotivated). These strategies have been particularly helpful in alleviating depression and anxiety.[66] Behavioral activation strategies focus on helping clients enhance daily activities and behaviors (eg, take a walk, go to the grocery store) so they receive the positive benefits of such participation (eg, feeling of accomplishment, kitchen full of necessary foods). In general, behavioral

**Table 2**
**Responding affirmatively to trans-specific discrimination**

| Sample Scenarios | Response Strategies to Avoid | Response Strategies to Embrace |
|---|---|---|
| Client reports people stared and laughed while grocery shopping | Universalize experiences of discrimination: "Everyone gets stared at sometimes" | Acknowledge and validate feelings: "It must be painful to be stared and gawked at when you are just trying to go about your day" |
| Client reports being systematically ignored by a professor | Search for alternative reasons for the perpetrator's behavior: "Have you considered that maybe he just didn't see your hand raised?" | Honor client resilience: "It is a testament to your strength that you continue to get up and go to class each day prepared to do your best even though your professor behaves that way toward you" |
| Client reports that once she started presenting as female at work she was told she must use the private restroom in the Human Resources office (a separate building) rather than the multistall women's restroom in her own office building | Minimize the consequences of discriminatory behavior: "Perhaps this is a good thing because you get to use the cleaner restroom with more privacy" | Recognize and attend to the emotional and other consequences of discriminatory treatment: "I can tell how isolating and ostracizing it feels for you to be the only one not allowed to use the restrooms in your own building; how have you been handling this?" |
| Client shares his feelings that he has not been called back for second interviews for several jobs because potential employers noted that his legal name is not consistent with his gender presentation | Normalize transphobic discrimination: "Finding a good job is tough for many folks these days" | Acknowledge and name transphobic-specific barriers: "It feels really unfair and discouraging to you that you continue to be passed over for jobs because of other people's transphobic attitudes and hiring practices" |

activation is particularly helpful for clients who have become isolated, apathetic, and hopeless in response to depression or social anxiety.[66] In TA-CBT, behavioral activation strategies are often used to foster transgender-specific connection among individuals who are isolated and/or disconnected from the larger transgender community.

Because affirming a transgender identity through connections to others in the transgender community is increasingly recognized as critical to well-being,[38,39] supporting behavioral activation toward this end is an integral component of TA-CBT. However, for some transgender clients, anxiety, depression, and feelings of despair impede them from engaging in identity-affirming activities. Typical behavioral activation assignments include generating lists of positive activities, developing and using weekly charts to schedule activities and responsibilities, and tracking moods and emotions in response to engaging in new behaviors and activities.[65] In TA-CBT the focus is on identifying specific transgender-affirming behaviors, activities, and sources of support that can be integrated into clients' daily lives. In addition to, or instead of, a traditional pleasant activities list, TA-CBT clinicians therefore help their clients generate lists of trans-affirming people, places, and activities. **Table 3** provides examples of these resources. In addition to the traditional goals of behavioral activation, TA behavioral activation strategies are designed to develop client resiliency by strengthening social support networks, fostering a sense of connection to the transgender community, and creating opportunities for agency and self-advocacy.

There are several considerations when helping clients develop a feasible transgender-specific behavioral activation plan. Because some TGNC clients may be disconnected from transgender resources, it is important that TA-CBT clinicians have the requisite knowledge of local, regional, national, and online resources and sources of support. In addition, clinicians must be aware of and sensitive to any potential barriers to accessing transgender-specific support. In addition to exploring potential emotional barriers (eg, anxiety about meeting new people), clinicians may need to spend time exploring potential interpersonal barriers. For instance, a fear of being "outed" when accessing local resources may be of particular concern for some

**Table 3**
**Trans-affirming activities list**

| Transgender-affirming Activity | Examples |
| --- | --- |
| Schedule time with affirming people | • Facetime with a trans friend<br>• Coffee date with supportive ally<br>• Phone call with affirming family member |
| Visit trans-affirming places | • Attend local trans support group<br>• Spend time in LGBTQ-affirming neighborhoods<br>• Visit the local trans or LGBTQ community center |
| Schedule identity-affirming activities | • Spend time visiting trans-specific Facebook pages, blogs, YouTube channels<br>• Stream trans-specific movies or documentaries<br>• Read memoirs about other trans people<br>• Plan for and attend local, regional, or national trans-specific conferences or workshops |
| Engage in trans-specific community-building activities | • Join a local or regional transgender equality group and go to meetings<br>• Participate in the Trans Day of Silence, Trans Day of Remembrance, or Trans Day of Visibility Events |

*Abbreviation:* LGBTQ, lesbian, gay, bisexual, transgender, queer.

clients. Economic (eg, not having consistent transportation to attend events or groups) and logistical (eg, rural area) barriers also need to be considered and prospective solutions generated. Troubleshooting these challenges and developing a feasible plan for gradually increasing transgender-specific involvement at a pace that feels safe and comfortable for the client is important to the success of TA behavioral activation strategies.

## SUMMARY

Increasingly, TGNC individuals are taking steps to live authentically and the affirmation of their identities is recognized as critical to well-being. Nonetheless, TGNC individuals continue to be a highly marginalized population, subject to transphobia that manifests itself in the form of oppression, discrimination, victimization, and internalized stigma. Mental health clinicians must be prepared to help TGNC individuals manage minority stress and cope with the effects of traumatic events. TA-CBT enables mental health clinicians to do so by implementing CBT, a highly effective and widely used model for developing adaptive coping skills and reducing distress within a transgender-affirming clinical context. TA-CBT combines cognitive and behavioral techniques and strategies with an inclusive and affirmative understanding of transgender identities and experiences. TA-CBT validates the hardships experienced by transgender populations and enhances the support, resources, and skills necessary to effectively navigate interpersonal, social, and cultural contexts rooted in cisgender privilege.

## REFERENCES

1. Monro S. Beyond male and female: poststructuralism and the spectrum of gender. Int J Transgend 2005;8:3–22.
2. Saltzburg S, Davis TS. Co-authoring gender-queer youth identities: discursive tellings and retellings. J Ethn Cult Divers Soc Work 2010;19:87–108.
3. Austin A. "There I am": a grounded theory study of young adults navigating a transgender or gender nonconforming identity within a context of oppression and invisibility. Sex Roles 2016.
4. Grant JM, Mottet LA, Tanis J, et al. Injustice at every turn: a report of the National Transgender Discrimination Survey [Internet]. Washington, DC: National Center for Transgender Equality and National Gay and Lesbian Task Force; 2011. Available at: http://endtransdiscrimination.org/report.html. Accessed March 13, 2016.
5. Collazo A, Austin A, Craig SL. Facilitating transition among transgender clients: components of effective clinical practice. Clin Soc Work J 2013;41:228–37.
6. Austin A, Craig SL. Transgender affirmative cognitive behavioral therapy: clinical considerations and applications. Prof Psychol Res Pr 2015;46:21–9.
7. Austin A, Craig SL. Empirically supported interventions for sexual and gender minority youth. J Evid Inf Soc Work 2015;12:567–78.
8. Meyer IH. Prejudice, social stress, and mental health in lesbian, gay, and bisexual populations: conceptual issues and research evidence. Psychol Bull 2003;129: 674–97.
9. Bockting WO, Miner MH, Swinburne Romine RE, et al. Stigma, mental health, and resilience in an online sample of the US transgender population. Am J Public Health 2013;103:943–51.
10. Hendricks ML, Testa RJ. A conceptual framework for clinical work with transgender and gender nonconforming clients: an adaptation of the minority stress model. Prof Psychol Res Pr 2012;43:460–7.

11. Meyer IH. Resilience in the study of minority stress and health of sexual and gender minorities. Psychol Sex Orientat Gend Divers 2015;2:209–13.
12. Grossman AH, D'Augelli AR. Transgender youth and life-threatening behaviors. Suicide Life Threat Behav 2007;37:527–37.
13. Stotzer RL, Silverschanz P, Wilson A. Gender identity and social services: barriers to care. J Soc Serv Res 2013;39:63–77.
14. Goldblum P, Testa RJ, Pflum S, et al. The relationship between gender-based victimization and suicide attempts in transgender people. Prof Psychol Res Pr 2012;43:468–75.
15. Kosciw J, Greytak E, Palmer N, et al. GLESN National School Climate Survey. 2013. Available at: http://www.glsen.org/sites/default/files/2013%20National%20School%20Climate%20Survey%20Full%20Report_0.pdf. Accessed January 24, 2016.
16. Dragowski EA, Halkitis PN, Grossman AH, et al. Sexual orientation victimization and posttraumatic stress symptoms among lesbian, gay, and bisexual youth. J Gay Lesbian Soc Serv 2011;23:226–49.
17. Budge SL, Adelson JL, Howard KA. Anxiety and depression in transgender individuals: the roles of transition status, loss, social support, and coping. J Consult Clin Psychol 2013;81:545–57.
18. dickey LM, Reisner SL, Juntunen CL. Non-suicidal self-injury in a large online sample of transgender adults. Prof Psychol Res Pr 2015;46:3.
19. Nemoto T, Bödeker B, Iwamoto M. Social support, exposure to violence and transphobia, and correlates of depression among male-to-female transgender women with a history of sex work. Am J Public Health 2011;101:1980–8.
20. Nuttbrock L, Hwahng S, Bockting W, et al. Psychiatric impact of gender-related abuse across the life course of male-to-female transgender persons. J Sex Res 2010;47:12–23.
21. Clements-Nolle K, Marx R, Katz M. Attempted suicide among transgender persons: the influence of gender-based discrimination and victimization. J Homosex 2006;51:53–69.
22. Haas AP, Rodgers PL, Herman JL. Suicide attempts among transgender and gender non-conforming adults, finding of the National Transgender Discrimination Survey. Los Angeles (CA): American Foundation for Suicide Prevention and the Williams Institute; 2014. Available at: http://williamsinstitute.law.ucla.edu/wp-content/uploads/AFSP-Williams-Suicide-Report-Final.pdf. Accessed March 2, 2016.
23. Shipherd JC, Maguen S, Skidmore WC, et al. Potentially traumatic events in a transgender sample: frequency and associated symptoms. Traumatology 2011; 17:56–67.
24. Alessi EJ, Martin JI. Intersection between trauma and identity. In: Eckstrand KL, Potter J, editors. Trauma, resilience, and health promotion for LGBT patients: what every healthcare provider should know. New York: Springer. in press.
25. D'Augelli AR, Grossman AH, Starks MT. Childhood gender atypicality, victimization, and PTSD among lesbian, gay, and bisexual youth. J Interpers Violence 2006;21:1462–82.
26. Roberts AL, Rosario M, Corliss HL, et al. Elevated risk of posttraumatic stress in sexual minority youths: mediation by childhood abuse and gender nonconformity. Am J Public Health 2012;102:1587–93.
27. Alessi EJ, Meyer IH, Martin JI. PTSD and sexual orientation: an examination of Criterion A1 and non-Criterion A1 events. Psychol Trauma 2013;5:149–57.
28. Bryant-Davis T, Ocampo C. Racist incident-based trauma. Couns Psychol 2005; 33:479–500.

29. Root MP. Reconstructing the impact of trauma on personality development: a feminist perspective. In: Brown LS, Ballou MB, editors. Personality and psychopathology: feminist reappraisals. New York: Guilford; 1992. p. 229–66.

30. Burnes TR, Dexter MM, Richmond K, et al. The experiences of transgender survivors of trauma who undergo social and medical transition. Traumatology 2016; 22:75–84.

31. Richmond KA, Burnes T, Carroll K. Lost in trans-lation: interpreting systems of trauma for transgender clients. Traumatology 2012;18:45–57.

32. Felitti VJ, Anda RF, Nordenberg D, et al. Relationship of childhood abuse and household dysfunction to many of the leading causes of death in adults: the Adverse Childhood Experiences (ACE) study. Am J Prev Med 1998;14:245–58.

33. Herman JL. Trauma and recovery. New York: Basic Books; 1992.

34. Van der Kolk B. The body keeps the score: brain, mind, and body in the healing of trauma. New York: Penguin; 2014.

35. Sánchez FJ, Vilain E. Collective self-esteem as a coping resource for male-to-female transsexuals. J Couns Psychol 2009;56:202–9.

36. Simons L, Schrager SM, Clark LF, et al. Parental support and mental health among transgender adolescents. J Adolesc Health 2013;53:791–3.

37. Pflum SR, Testa RJ, Balsam KF, et al. Social support, trans community connectedness, and mental health symptoms among transgender and gender nonconforming adults. Psychol Sex Orientat Gend Divers 2015;2:281–6.

38. Barr SM, Budge SL, Adelson JL. Transgender community belongingness as a mediator between strength of transgender identity and well-being. J Couns Psychol 2016;63:87–97.

39. Testa RJ, Jimenez CL, Rankin S. Risk and resilience during transgender identity development: the effects of awareness and engagement with other transgender people on affect. J Gay Lesbian Ment Health 2014;18:31–46.

40. Austin A, Craig SL, Goodman R. Bridging efforts to enhance support for the transgender community: a grand challenge for social work. Paper presented at: Society for Social Work Research 20th Annual Conference. Washington DC, January 14-17, 2016.

41. Austin A, Goodman R. The impact of social connectedness and internalized transphobic stigma on self-esteem among transgender and gender nonconforming adults. J Homosex 2016. [Epub ahead of print].

42. Horvath KJ, Iantaffi A, Grey JA, et al. A review of the content and format of transgender-related webpages. Health Commun 2012;27:457–66.

43. Craig SL, McInroy L. You can form a part of yourself online: the influence of new media on identity development and coming out for LGBTQ youth. J Gay Lesbian Ment Health 2014;18:95–109.

44. Singh AA. Transgender youth of color and resilience: negotiating oppression and finding support. Sex Roles 2013;68:690–702.

45. Newman PA, Fantus S. A social ecology of bias-based bullying of sexual and gender minority youth: toward a conceptualization of conversion bullying. J Gay Lesbian Soc Serv 2015;27:46–63.

46. Substance Abuse and Mental Health Services Administration. Ending conversion therapy: supporting and affirming LGBTQ youth [Internet]. Rockville (MD): Substance Abuse and Mental Health Services Administration; 2015. HHS Publication No. (SMA) 15-4928. Available at: http://store.samhsa.gov/shin/content/SMA15-4928/SMA15-4928.pdf. Accessed January 20, 2016.

47. Horn SS. Attitudes about sexual orientation. In: Patterson C, D'Augelli A, editors. Handbook of psychology and sexual orientation. Oxford: Oxford University Press; 2012. p. 229, 239–51.

48. Craig SL, Austin A, Alessi E. Gay affirmative cognitive behavioral therapy for sexual minority youth: a clinical adaptation and approach. Clin Soc Work J 2013;41: 258–66.

49. American Academy of Pediatrics Committee on Adolescence. Position paper: office-based care for lesbian, gay, bisexual, transgender, and questioning youth. Pediatrics 2013;132:198–203.

50. Hedman E, El Alaoui S, Lindefors N, et al. Clinical effectiveness and cost-effectiveness of Internet- vs. group-based cognitive behavior therapy for social anxiety disorder: 4-year follow-up of a randomized trial. Behav Res Ther 2014; 59:20–9.

51. Hofmann SG, Asnaani A, Vonk IJ, et al. The efficacy of cognitive behavioral therapy: a review of meta-analyses. Cognit Ther Res 2012;36:427–40.

52. Cary CE, McMillen JC. The data behind the dissemination: a systematic review of trauma-focused cognitive behavioral therapy for use with children and youth. Child Youth Serv Rev 2012;34:748–57.

53. Morley KC, Sitharthan G, Haber PS, et al. The efficacy of an opportunistic cognitive behavioral intervention package (OCB) on substance use and comorbid suicide risk: a multisite randomized controlled trial. J Consult Clin Psychol 2014;82:130.

54. Twomey C, O'Reilly G, Byrne M. Effectiveness of cognitive behavioural therapy for anxiety and depression in primary care: a meta-analysis. Fam Pract 2015; 32:3–15.

55. Beck A. Cognitive therapy: nature and relation to behavior therapy. Behav Ther 1970;1:184–200.

56. Beck JS. Cognitive behavior therapy: basics and beyond. New York: Guilford Press; 2011.

57. Mizock L, Mueser K. Employment, mental health, internalized stigma, and coping with transphobia among transgender individuals. Psychol Sex Orientat Gend Divers 2014;1:146–58.

58. Craig SL, Austin A. The AFFIRM open pilot feasibility study: a brief affirmative cognitive behavioral coping skills group intervention for sexual and gender minority youth. Child Youth Serv Rev 2016;64:136–44.

59. Winters K, Ehrbar RD. Beyond conundrum: strategies for diagnostic harm reduction. J Gay Lesbian Ment Health 2010;14:130–8.

60. Vaid-Menon A. Greater transgender visibility hasn't helped nonbinary people like me. Guardian 2015. Available at: http://www.theguardian.com/commentisfree/2015/oct/13/greater-transgender-visibility-hasnt-helped-nonbinary-people-like-me. Accessed February 7, 2016.

61. Payne P, Levine PA, Crane-Godreau MA. Somatic experiencing: using interoception and proprioception as core elements of trauma therapy. Front Psychol 2015; 6:93.

62. Davis M, Eshelman ER, McKay M. The relaxation and stress reduction workbook. Oakland (CA): New Harbinger Publications; 2008.

63. Leahy RL. Cognitive therapy techniques: a practitioner's guide. New York: Guilford Press; 2003.

64. Padesky CA, Mooney KA. Strengths-based cognitive–behavioural therapy: a four-step model to build resilience. Clin Psychol Psychother 2012;19:283–90.

65. Martell CR, Safren SA, Prince SE. Cognitive-behavioral therapies with lesbian, gay, and bisexual clients. New York: Guilford Press; 2004.

66. Hopko DR, Ryba MM, McIndoo C, et al. Behavioral activation. In: Nezu AM, Nezu CM, editors. The Oxford handbook of cognitive and behavioral therapies. New York: Oxford University Press. in press.

# Group Psychotherapy with Transgender and Gender Nonconforming Adults

## Evidence-Based Practice Applications

Nicholas C. Heck, PhD

## KEYWORDS

- Affirmative psychotherapy • Gender identity • Group therapy • Mental health
- Transgender

## KEY POINTS

- Research evaluating the effectiveness of group psychotherapy interventions with transgender and gender nonconforming (TGNC) clients has yet to be conducted.
- Counseling competencies, standards of care, and practice guidelines are available to assist mental health professionals working with TGNC clients within group settings.
- Mental health professionals should adopt an affirmative approach to the practice of group psychotherapy with TGNC clients.
- Integrating psychoeducation, affect regulation, cognitive coping, and problem-solving skills may be beneficial for TGNC clients receiving group psychotherapy.

As the field of psychology pushes further into the twenty-first century, there is a growing awareness that not as much is known as should be about how well psychotherapeutic services meet the needs of diverse populations. This is especially true for people who identify as transgender and/or express gender variance beyond the confines of the socially constructed gender binary. Questions pertaining to the acceptability and effectiveness of interventions for TGNC clients remain largely unanswered. Recent systematic reviews reveal that TGNC identities are rarely, if ever, reported in psychotherapy trials for anxiety and depression; such identities are also under-reported in substance abuse research.[1,2] Studies examining the acceptability and efficacy of therapeutic interventions and modalities, such as group psychotherapy, for use with TGNC persons have yet to be conducted. Although there have been recent efforts to adapt and evaluate existing evidence-based interventions for gay and bisexual men,[3] such efforts are nonexistent for TGNC persons. Furthermore, the competence of mental health

The author has no relevant financial interests pertaining to this article.
Department of Psychology, Marquette University, Cramer Hall, 323, PO Box 1881, Milwaukee, WI 53201, USA
*E-mail address:* nicholas.heck@marquette.edu

professionals with respect to their ability to meet the needs of TGNC clients, although likely improving, is less than ideal.[4] There is much work to be done to ensure that TGNC people can access appropriate and effective mental health services.

Recently, psychotherapy researchers have begun to describe how to tailor existing evidence-based interventions for use in group counseling to meet the needs of TGNC persons. For example, Austin and Craig[5] describe an 8-session cognitive-behavioral approach for TGNC clients that could be adapted for the group modality. Dickey and Loewy[6] discuss important considerations for providing group psychotherapy services to TGNC clients from a social justice perspective. Heck and colleagues[7] describe the process of developing a time-limited, experiential/process therapy group for TGNC clients and the key themes that emerge over the course of the group. Menvielle and Rodnan[8] also describe an assessment and treatment program for TGNC adolescents; their article includes a thematic review of the topics that often arise in their therapy group for the parents of TGNC adolescents.

Early scholarship devoted to the topic of group psychotherapy with TGNC clients relied heavily on descriptive reports. Until more psychotherapy outcome and evaluation research is conducted, it remains unclear which interventions and modalities work best for reducing distress and promoting positive health outcomes for TGNC people. Despite this nascent state of the affairs, hopefully mental health professionals who work with TGNC clients will use evidence-based interventions where appropriate as well as nonspecific therapeutic factors that contribute to the effectiveness of psychotherapy.[9] Nonspecific therapeutic factors are therapeutic elements (eg, acceptance, empathy, warmth, and therapeutic alliance) that are found in most therapies regardless of a therapist's theoretic orientation.[9,10] According to Alan Malyon,[11] a pioneer in the psychosocial treatment of gay men and lesbian women, 1 nonspecific factor that is thought especially important is that of therapist affirmation. Malyon[11] advocates that therapists affirm their clients' same-sex sexual orientation to counter past instances of invalidation and homophobia. The concept of affirmative psychotherapy has now been widely adapted for use with TGNC clients.[12,13] Affirmative counseling and psychotherapy for TGNC clients is culturally relevant, addresses the influence of social inequities, enhances resilience and fosters coping, and reduces systematic barriers experienced by TGNC people.[14] With the concept of affirmative psychotherapy in mind, the purpose of this article is to review the group psychotherapy literature, highlighting competencies required to offer group psychotherapy services to TGNC clients and to describe interventions that are especially relevant for TGNC clients.

## MAKING THE CASE FOR GROUP PSYCHOTHERAPY WITH TRANSGENDER AND GENDER NONCONFORMING CLIENTS

Group psychotherapy is an especially appropriate treatment modality for TGNC clients for several reasons. First, although not specific to TGNC clients, several randomized controlled trials and meta-analytic studies demonstrate the general efficacy of the group modality for a range of psychosocial challenges.[15–17] Research also shows that the group modality produces treatment effects that are often similar to those derived from individual therapy.[18] Second, group therapy is a cost-effective treatment approach, which is an important consideration given that TGNC people may experience economic marginalization.[19] Third, group therapy provides opportunities for TGNC clients to develop genuine and gratifying interpersonal relationships, which is important given that TGNC people often experience isolation.[19] Finally, group therapies often include several nonspecific therapeutic factors that are likely to promote authentic personal growth and development.

Yalom and Leszcz[20] identify 11 therapeutic factors that are critical to the success of group therapy: instillation of hope, universality, imparting information, altruism, corrective reenactment of critical relationship dynamics, socialization, imitative behavior, interpersonal learning, cohesion, catharsis, and existential influences. Although a discussion of each therapeutic factor as it relates to group work with TGNC clients is beyond the scope of this article, these factors remain relevant. For example, many transgender people experience discomfort and distress related to the incongruence between their sex and gender, often suffering in isolation.[21] Thus, the therapeutic factor of universality, a process in which group members begin to see themselves and their challenges reflected in the experiences and identities of the other members,[20] is especially relevant. Additionally, an increased sense of universality may foster more positive feelings about and a greater sense of connection to the TGNC community. Such feelings and connectedness are important to promote because they are associated with lower levels of psychological distress and suicidality among TGNC people.[22,23]

Another important therapeutic factor is interpersonal learning, which occurs when a group member displays a maladaptive interpersonal behavior, receives feedback from the group about the behavior, internalizes the feedback, learns a new behavior that replaces the maladaptive behavior, and receives additional feedback that increases the likelihood that the new behavior will be displayed again in the future.[20] As TGNC group members are encountering new ways to explore and express their identities, the process of interpersonal learning provides opportunities to receive feedback that can shape how members view and express themselves. This feedback and shaping process can enhance self-understanding and promote authenticity in ways that are conducive to developing and maintaining interpersonal relationships. Furthermore, interpersonal learning can help TGNC group members express their emotions about past experiences of invalidation in ways that foster intimacy and help them connect with other individuals who can provide support and validation. Interpersonal learning can enhance self-understanding and provide TGNC group members with cathartic opportunities. These experiences are often rated by group members as the most beneficial aspects of psychotherapy groups.[24,25]

## GROUP THERAPY PRACTICE GUIDELINES AND COMPETENCIES FOR USE WITH TRANSGENDER AND GENDER NONCONFORMING CLIENTS

Several professional bodies have offered guidance for mental health professionals who work with TGNC clients. For example, the World Professional Association for Transgender Health publishes *Standards of Care for the Health of Transsexual, Transgender, and Gender Nonconforming People*,[26] which provides clinical guidance to both mental health and medical providers to assist them in their work to help TGNC people find lasting satisfaction and comfort with their identity and health. The *SOC* identifies group psychotherapy as a therapeutic option for TGNC individuals experiencing gender dysphoria, mental health concerns, and social isolation; however, the *SOC* does not provide recommendations about the kinds of interventions that should be included as part of a group psychotherapy service.

The American Psychological Association Task Force "Guidelines for Psychological Practice with Transgender and Gender Nonconforming People" assist mental health professionals as they work to provide affirmative psychotherapy services.[4] The Task Force offers 16 guidelines organized into 5 clusters:

1. Foundational knowledge and awareness
2. Stigma, discrimination, and barriers to treatment

3. Life span development
4. Assessment and intervention
5. Research, education, and training

Mental health professionals who wish to build their competence to deliver services to TGNC clients should have a working knowledge of and familiarity with the *SOC* and the American Psychological Association guidelines.

The American Counseling Association (ACA) "Competencies for Counseling Transgender Clients"[27] include 103 competencies that coincide with the 8 training domains specified by the Council for Accreditation of Counseling and Related Educational Programs. Within the area of group psychotherapy, 16 therapist competencies are identified (**Table 1**). This discussion addresses these competencies in conjunction with the stages of group psychotherapy outlined by Yalom and Leszcz.[24] Although certain competencies are discussed in relation to specific group stages, mental health professionals should be mindful of all of the ACA competencies in their work with TGNC clients and not unnecessarily rule out the relevance of additional competencies for particular group stages.

Group leaders must continually monitor and assess their own biases and countertransference responses throughout all phases of group work with TGNC clients (as specified by competencies D.14. and D.15.). Thus, leaders should have self-awareness of their own biases and be aware of how their own gender identities, beliefs about gender, and knowledge (or lack thereof) may have an impact on the group. Group leaders should be comfortable asking for and listening to feedback about how their own gender identities may have an impact on group dynamics. Group leaders should encourage group members to reflect on this in the present moment and in the future, especially if they find themselves experiencing negative emotions related to the group leader(s). When group leaders are cisgender, especially when they are cisgender men, it is especially important to solicit feedback about how cisgender and male privilege have an impact on the group and the member-leader relationships. It is important for group leaders to recognize such power differentials, empathizing with and validating the emotions of group members as they share challenges that occur in their everyday lives.[7]

### Pregroup Planning

#### Therapist preparation

Before initiating group work with TGNC clients, mental health professionals must ensure that they are aware of their own biases and countertransference issues, especially those related to diverse identities (and the intersections of these identities) that are likely reflected among the group members (eg, ethnicity, gender, and sexual orientation). As specified by competencies D.14. and D.15., they must be aware of how their own gender identities and biases may have an impact on group dynamics and seek consultation or supervision to minimize the likelihood of their biases negatively affecting the group. Mental health professionals must also possess the knowledge and skills necessary to offer a psychotherapy group (as specified by competency D.16.). Unfortunately, mental health professionals may find it challenging to acquire the foundational knowledge and supervision necessary for serving TGNC clients using the group modality. Professional conferences are beginning to offer more continuing education programming, however, devoted to transgender health care topics, as are academic centers devoted to transgender health. For example, the Center of Excellence for Transgender Health at the University of California, San Francisco (http://www.transhealth.ucsf.edu), offers an online learning course to assist clinical

**Table 1**
**American Counseling Association competencies for counseling with transgender clients—section D: group work**

| Section | Description |
|---------|-------------|
| D.1. | Maintain a nonjudgmental, supportive stance on all expressions of gender identity and sexuality and establish this as a standard for group members as well. |
| D.2. | Facilitate group members' understanding that mental health professionals' attempts to change a member's gender identity (eg, conversion or reparative therapies) are not supported by research and, moreover, may have life-threatening consequences. |
| D.3. | Involve members in establishing the group treatment plans, expectations, and goals, which should be reviewed periodically throughout the group. These should foster the safety and inclusion of transgender members. |
| D.4. | Provide education and opportunities for social learning about a wide array of choices regarding coming out and transitioning if indicated or warranted. |
| D.5. | Recognize the impact of power, privilege, and oppression within the group, especially among the counselor and members and between members of advantaged and marginalized groups. |
| D.6. | Consider diversity (ie, gender identity, sex assigned at birth, sexual orientation, mental and physical ability status, mental health concerns, race, ethnicity, religion, and socioeconomic class) when selecting and screening group members and be sensitive to how these diverse identities may affect group dynamics. |
| D.7. | Be aware of the unique status of an individual who is the only transgender group member, and create a safe space in which that person can share her/his experiences if feeling comfortable. In this case, it is especially important to foster a sense of security through the use of respectful language toward the transgender member (eg, correct pronouns and names and gender-affirmative terminology of transition interventions). |
| D.8. | In gender-specific groups (eg, inpatient treatment settings and substance abuse treatment), transgender individuals need to attend the gender group with which they identify (instead of the gender group that they were assigned at birth). |
| D.9. | Acknowledge the impact of institutionalized and personalized transphobia on transgender members' comfort with disclosing and reflecting on their experiences that occur inside and outside of group. |
| D.10. | Actively intervene when either overt or covert hostility toward transgender-identified members threatens group security and cohesion. This applies to both transgender-specific groups and any group that has transgender members. |
| D.11. | Recognize that although group support can be helpful, peer pressure to conform to specific expression or plan of action exists within the group. |
| D.12. | Coordinate treatment with other professionals working with transgender members, while maintaining confidentiality within the group. |
| D.13. | Refer clients to other mental and physical health services when either initiated by the group member or due to clinical judgment that the member is in need of these interventions. |
| D.14. | Be aware of how their own gender identities, beliefs about gender, and lack of knowledge about transgender issues may affect group processes. |
| D.15. | Seek consultation or supervision to ensure that the counselor's potential biases and knowledge deficits do not negatively affect group dynamics. |
| D.16. | Ideally have previous experience working with transgender individuals in both non–transgender-specific and transgender-specific groups. If no previous counseling experience with transgender individuals exists, consultation and supervision with mental health professionals who are competent and have more experience working with transgender issues is even more critical. |

*From* Burnes TR, Singh AA, Harper AJ, et al. American Counseling Association competencies for counseling with transgender clients. Journal Of LGBT Issues In Counseling 2010;4:135-9; with permission.

staff and providers in fostering an affirming environment for TGNC clients. Furthermore, Heck and colleagues[7] identify key articles and texts used to train leaders of a transgender-specific therapy group and offer suggestions for locating appropriate supervision for those already in practice but lacking the necessary competence to offer a group.

Even if mental health professionals have the requisite training to work with TGNC clients, many may lack awareness of the specific challenges associated with conducting a transgender-specific group because TGNC persons are often invisible within communities and little is known about their mental and medical health service needs. Therefore, it is necessary for mental health professionals to advocate for and, whenever possible, include this population in formal needs assessments. Mental health professionals should network within their communities by connecting with local lesbian, gay, bisexual, and transgender (LGBT) community centers and state organizations that advocate for LGBT issues to determine what, if any, mental and physical health services are available for TGNC people. To determine whether there is a sufficient referral base of clients to establish a group, mental health professionals can consult with colleagues in their communities to identify potential group members, some of whom may already be engaged in individual therapy. If it is challenging to obtain the critical mass necessary to form a TGNC-specific therapy group, mental health professionals can expand the group offering to include multifamily group services. Menvielle and Rodnan[8] describe a group therapy service for the parents of transgender adolescents; key themes addressed within the group include processing emotional reactions to the adolescent's TGNC identity, coming out to relatives and friends, navigating loss or grief, coping with stress and challenges associated with the transition process, and discussing fears about the adolescent's safety and health.[8]

### Addressing systemic issues

Before starting a therapy group for TGNC clients, mental health professionals may need to address systemic issues within practice settings to ensure compliance with the ACA competencies. For example, intake paperwork may require modification to ensure gender inclusivity, such that clients are asked to write in their gender on a blank line; many commonly used psychological tests are not gender inclusive and thus also require modification.[28] Clinics should also offer gender-neutral restrooms, and inpatient units should provide rooming accommodations that are sensitive to the needs of TGNC clients rather than those based on a client's sex assigned at birth. Competency D.8. indicates that in gender-specific groups, TGNC clients are to attend a group with which they identify rather than a group that coincides with the sex they were assigned at birth. These changes can be challenging to enact within inpatient and larger hospital settings because there may be broader systemic policies that require modification to ensure that staff members are aware of, knowledgeable about, and committed to meeting the unique needs of TGNC clients. Also, within these settings it is not uncommon to have a group that contains only 1 TGNC client. When this occurs, group leaders must consider how to ensure the safety and security of the TGNC group member (competency D.7.). It is important to discuss the appropriate use of pronouns and for the leaders to express their commitment to ensuring that the group is affirming of gender diversity. Overall, such advocacy and educational efforts are important, especially when carried out by cisgender professionals who can leverage their privilege in these settings and reduce the burden on TGNC clients and staff, who are too often forced to call attention to institutional barriers.[14]

### Logistical decision making

Dickey and Loewy[6] offer guidance to answer questions that typically confront mental health professionals who are preparing to offer group psychotherapy services specifically for TGNC clients. Examples of such questions might include the following: What type of group should be offered? Should the group adopt an open, closed, and/or time-limited format? Where should the group meet? Should the group comprise trans men, trans women, people who identify as genderqueer, and/or people who are cisgender?

With respect to the type of group, mental health professionals need to determine whether they should offer a support group or a therapy/process group. Although there are numerous distinctions between support and therapy/process groups, one difference involves how to address subgrouping or out-of-group encounters among group members. Typically, support groups do not attempt to prohibit out-of-group encounters and may actually encourage such opportunities for socialization. Within therapy groups, especially those that emphasize interpersonal processes/dynamics, reducing the potential for subgrouping helps ensure that the group process is contained within the group sessions.[7,20] Thus, mental health professionals should carefully balance the potential detriments to group functioning that can stem from subgrouping with the potential benefits that may come from out-of-group socialization. In either case, the issue of subgrouping should be considered and discussed early in the group to determine the members' preferences for navigating this issue.

Another consideration involves whether to offer an open (ie, new members are added over time) or closed (ie, new members are not typically added after the first 2–3 sessions) group and whether the group is time limited or will continue indefinitely.[20] Open groups tend to tolerate changes in membership when the group leader remains consistent, which may not be possible in certain settings where turnover is high or therapists rotate through multiple clinics. An open group may be preferable when the leader remains constant and there is a sufficient referral base to repopulate the group when members terminate. Offering a closed and time-limited (ie, 12, 16, or 20 weeks) group can help ensure that all members are working together to achieve their goals within a similar time fame. With respect to location, mental health professionals must consider the safety of the group members. The venue should also be conveniently located, accessible, affirming of transgender people, and private. Taken together, private clinics and LGBT community centers may be ideal locations. In addition, public hospitals and religious/spiritual venues that are LGBT affirming might also offer meeting space rented at little or no cost to the group.[6]

Competency D.6. indicates that group leaders consider the composition of the therapy group with respect to characteristics of the group members and be mindful of how a group's composition may have an impact on the group dynamics. For example, Dickey and Loewy[6] reported concerns over attrition at transgender support groups, specifically for trans men. They noted the disproportionate number of trans women, relative to trans men, in their groups, and attrition was attributed to the unique needs of the trans men not receiving adequate attention. This highlights the importance of selecting group members, whenever possible, to create a balanced group (eg, having at least 2 trans men or 2 pre/post-transition members) where members share a sense of universality in their goals and identities. Even within balanced groups, it is important that group leaders effectively manage and structure the sessions to ensure that the needs of all group members receive attention. In groups that are unbalanced with respect to specific participant characteristics, leaders would be wise to identify similarities in the lived experiences of group members in advance of the first group session. A pregroup consultation meeting can facilitate this process by allowing group leaders to identify such experiences, while also helping potential group members

Identify goals and possible challenges that might compromise the group or an individual member's likelihood of having a successful group experience.[7] Group leaders can then draw on the information obtained within the consultation session in an effort to foster connections among group members by facilitating conversations that reveal these similarities and commonalities.

### The Initial Stage

In the initial stage, group members are tasked with trying to understand how they will use the group experience to achieve their goals and develop connections with other members who make attending group sessions a pleasurable and rewarding experience.[20] The leader is tasked with calming anxieties, establishing ground rules, providing psychoeducation, and insuring that group members identify their goals for the group. Group leaders may also find it helpful to introduce problem-solving skills during the initial stage.

### Establishing ground rules

Once the logistics of a group are established and group members identified, the initial group session offers the first opportunity to see how the group functions as a whole. Because anxieties are often higher at first group meetings, group leaders are wise to provide structure while acknowledging that future groups may be less structured (as in the case of process groups). In accordance with competencies D.1., D.2., D.12., and D.13., group leaders may wish to consider establishing a list of rights for transgender group members that can function as a means of addressing specific competencies and facilitating the process of establishing ground rules for the group. **Box 1** contains

---

**Box 1**
**Rights and responsibilities of transgender and gender nonconforming group members**

- Members have the right to freely express their gender identity and sexuality without judgment.

- Members have the right to share their experiences with the group without concern that their statements will be disclosed outside the group by other group members.

- Members have the right to receive coordinated care, wherein the group leaders communicate with other mental health and medical professionals to help ensure that the members receive quality health care services.

- Members have the right to request and be provided with referrals for additional mental, physical, and other health or transition-related services.

- Members are responsible for treating one another, the leader, and clinic staff with respect.

- Members are responsible for arriving on time for all group sessions.

- Members are responsible for attending all group sessions or informing the group leader at the onset of the group of any planned absences.

- Members are responsible for maintaining the confidentiality of the group; what happens in group should not be discussed outside the group. Members should also refrain from discussing group members who are no longer part of the group.

- Members are responsible for cleaning up after themselves when using the clinic restrooms to prepare for the group (eg, dressing and applying makeup or other products).

- Members are responsible for completing any homework or out-of-group activities that are assigned during the group.

- Members are expected to attend sessions free from the influence of substances.

an example of a list of rights that might be presented to group members with an invitation to develop their own and/or modify this list. During this conversation, group leaders can address the issue of conversion/reparative therapies and articulate the problems inherent with such efforts. This conversation also offers an opportunity to discuss the importance and limits of confidentiality, which is critical to creating a safe group environment.[7]

## Psychoeducation

During the initial stages of groups, leaders also have an opportunity to provide psychoeducation about common mental health concerns and interpersonal challenges that are experienced by TGNC people. Group leaders can then begin to facilitate conversations that help illuminate how the therapy group can help to address these concerns and challenges. Such conversations also lay the foundation for providing psychoeducation about the impact of minority stress on the health of TGNC people. Recent research and scholarship suggests that mental health professionals should help TGNC clients understand the concept of minority stress as it relates to health disparities that have an impact on TGNC people.[5,29] Meyer's minority stress model[30] identifies 4 stress processes that seem to capture many of the stressors experienced by TGNC people (ie, experiencing prejudice, expecting prejudice, concealment, and internalizing transphobia).[31] When understood by group members, this framework can help them recognize that current and past experiences of psychological distress are often attributable to the higher rates of stress that TGNC people are exposed to in their everyday lives. Thus group leaders can work to help members distinguish general forms of stress from transgender-specific minority stressors. Such discussions also provide opportunities to foster universality and instill hope that TGNC clients can learn coping skills in group therapy to help them manage the challenges associated with life in contexts that are often unwelcoming.

## Identifying goals

Once the ground rules and logistical aspects of the group are established, group leaders want to facilitate conversations about individual goals and/or treatment plans, which is consistent with competency D.3. As group members come to realize that they share many of the same goals, a sense of universality and collective responsibility begins to emerge, which in turn helps foster connections among members. Group members who have previously transitioned and/or those who experience their gender identity in a more established manner may see themselves reflected in the current goals of members who have only recently come to realize that they are TGNC. There are also opportunities for group members who have a more established sense of their gender identities to learn from other members who may express their gender identities in novel ways using technology and resources that have not been available in the past.

Group leaders should also remember that TGNC people seek therapy for challenges that are both distally and proximally related to their gender identities. Goals that are more proximally related to a member's gender identity likely coincide with the member's gender identity development. Lev's[21] developmental approach can be an especially helpful resource for group therapists as they begin the process of helping group members identify and refine their personal goals for the group. Lev's model, entitled "transgender emergence," comprises 6 stages (ie, awareness, seeking information/reaching out, disclosure, identity exploration, transition considerations, and integration), with each stage having specific therapeutic tasks. Although stage models have often been the subject of critique, especially when rigidly applied, group leaders can consider the stages and accompanying therapeutic tasks to ensure that the group

~~sessions include content and other sessions that are especially relevant to the individual~~ members. The model can also help group leaders foreshadow tasks that are on the horizon and return to topics that may have been avoided or remain unaddressed.

### Problem solving

Problem solving in psychotherapy involves techniques, discussions, or activities that allow an individual to develop a systematic method for solving problems.[32] Research suggests that facilitating an orientation toward problem solving and teaching specific problem-solving skills can be beneficial for people experiencing psychosocial challenges.[32,33] As group members discuss their challenges, group leaders see opportunities to introduce this skill, which typically involves problem identification, possible solution generation, the evaluation of pros and cons, and taking action. As group members become more adept at engaging in problem solving, group leaders can shift the focus beyond teaching the basic steps of problem solving to discussing the process of addressing such concerns. For example, group leaders can obtain input from peers with similar experiences, celebrate achievements, receive support in the event that efforts to resolve a particular problem are thwarted, and address maladaptive interpersonal behaviors within the here-and-now of the group. The case of Jack (a pseudonym) helps illustrate the use of STEPS,[34] a specific approach to problem solving:

> Jack, a middle-class, white trans man of Dutch and Irish ancestry in his late 30s, repeatedly expressed frustration about how his finances were preventing him from having a subcutaneous mastectomy (top surgery). The first time this frustration was voiced, the group leader solicited reactions from the group members, who provided empathy by sharing similar experiences. Other group members shared their experiences with overcoming such challenges by carefully budgeting their expenses and looking for ways to save and reallocate money. Hearing a discrete problem and potential methods to address it, the group leader used this situation as an opportunity to introduce the STEPS approach to problem-solving, wherein clients are instructed to (1) state the problem, (2) think of possible solutions, (3) evaluate the pros/cons of each possible solution, (4) pick a possible solution and try it out, and (5) see if the problem is resolved. The group discussed how it can be difficult to engage in structured problem solving due to the sheer number of problems they face. Eventually they acknowledged that using a structured process can be helpful for solving problems, especially if, over time, the problem-solving process replaces rumination about problems and occurs somewhat automatically.

> In a subsequent session, Jack again expressed frustration about this problem. The group members provided empathy but also were curious as to what plans Jack had put into place to try to resolve the issue. When Jack confessed that he had not thought about it after the previous group, the leader again provided empathy and encouraged Jack to consider working through the problem-solving method as an out-of-group activity.

> At the next session, Jack was asked how this had gone, and he again reported not giving the issue much thought outside the group. Noticing that the group members were becoming frustrated, the group leader shifted the conversation toward the topic of goal setting, wherein the surgery was identified as a long-term goal, with short-term and medium-term goals that would lead to achieving the long-term goal also being identified. Once this occurred and a simple short-term goal was identified, Jack returned to the group and reported that he set up an automatic, monthly money transfer from his checking account to a savings account.

*As a next step, Jack decided that his next goal would be to read about the different types of surgeries and begin compiling a list of surgeons and their surgical specialties. Although Jack was working toward addressing this problem, he continued to express financial concerns at subsequent group meetings.*

The case of Jack highlights how a structured approach to solving problems can be integrated into the group setting. It also highlights how problem solving can be linked to goal setting in a way that can help reframe problems as goals to be achieved. Finally, Jack's case highlights the importance of group leaders' skills in implementing interventions in a flexible manner, while also being attuned to interpersonal/process dynamics that evolve over multiple sessions. Although Jack's initial problem seems resolved, his continued focus on finances likely warrant additional exploration to better understand the function of this behavior and help Jack come to understand how his frustrations have an impact on those around him.

### The Second Stage

During the second stage, members begin to establish their roles within the group and a social hierarchy starts to emerge; through this process, conflicts between members and with the group leader may arise.[20] Additionally, members may begin to question their values and the values of one another. Group leaders must be able to detect conflict, help members understand the origins of conflict, foster insight, and illuminate interpersonal process dynamics.

#### Addressing conflicts

Group leaders should be attuned to subtle signs that the group is or individual members are applying pressures to conform to unspoken norms and outdated expectations about coming out and/or transitioning. Competencies D.10 and D.11. address the capacity for group leaders to actively intervene when overt or covert hostilities toward TGNC group members threaten the group and individual members. Such pressure and hostilities may be most evident when group members, especially those who transitioned when the *SOC* was more rigid, interact with other group members who are currently transitioning and perhaps have more flexibility in how they navigate the transition process and the multitude of decisions that are embedded in this process.[7] Conflicts may also arise when group members express their gender in ways that challenge societal norms, elect not to pursue certain transition-related procedures/services, or engage in illegal activities. In such situations, group leaders should gently explore the origins of the group members' beliefs about the behaviors or decisions that give rise to conflicts in an effort to foster greater insight, understanding, and acceptance of individual member's decisions and experiences. Reframing conflicts as opportunities to genuinely express care and concern for one another in a nonjudgmental manner can foster connection and diffuse tension within the group.

#### Conflicting values

As the group matures, it is often the case that the values of group members may be questioned and become amenable to change. This process can cause emotional discomfort, however, for individual members and the group as a whole. Thus, it is incumbent on the group leaders to recognize this process and illuminate it for the group. Hayes and colleagues[35] acknowledge that although values are socialized, individuals ultimately are free to choose their values. The process of socialization, especially in communities and families who are transphobic, can result in TGNC people attempting to live their lives in accordance with values that conflict with their gender identities. Ambivalence and conflict arise when socialized values are incongruent with a core part of an individual group member's identity. This can result in individuals attempting to suppress certain components of their identities, ongoing conflict, or resolution though the discovery and adoption of new values.

Consider a situation in which a trans woman, who has yet to come out to her adult children and begin living fulltime as a woman, expresses fears about losing her family and a desire to continue in her role as a loving husband and father. In this instance, a conflict may exist between the value of authenticity and the value of being a loving husband and father. There are also legitimate fears about rejection and abandonment that contribute to her distress. Using the group, leaders can help the client address her fears and begin to resolve the ambivalence she experiences. The group leader can use Socratic questioning to separate the 2 issues so that each can be addressed individually. Then the leader can use the group to discern what it means to be loving, to be a husband, to be a father, and to be authentic, which may help the client recognize that the behaviors underlying specific values can persist, even if the value is altered. This can help the client separate the conflict she experiences with respect to her values from fears she has about experiencing abandonment and rejection from her family. Once separated, these issues may become more manageable, such that each can be explored within the context of the other members' experiences.

### The Third Stage

The third stage of the group begins as conflicts resolve and the group members become more adept at recognizing patterns of interpersonal behaviors that serve to foster or impede the development of cohesion.[20] The leader is tasked with fostering and helping to maintain cohesion while also assisting members as they confront and work to overcome the effects oppression, prejudice, and internalized transphobia. Promoting learned agency, affect regulation, and cognitive coping may help members navigate these challenges.

### Fostering and maintaining cohesiveness

Cohesiveness in group therapy represents the quality of the individual group members' relationships with one another, with the group leader(s), and with the group as a whole; members of cohesive groups feel warmth, safety, comfort, and connectedness within the group.[20] Group cohesion is an essential nonspecific therapeutic factor that is strongly and consistently associated with positive outcomes.[36] Thus, a critical goal for group leaders is to foster and maintain cohesiveness.

To attain this goal, group leaders must assist the group members as they take interpersonal risks, engage in self-disclosure, and openly express emotions. Fostering cohesiveness can be accomplished by creating situations where members are able to share in a group experience. Competency D.4. specifies that group members should provide opportunities for learning about a wide range of choices relating to coming out and transition processes. Group leaders should consider how to address this competency above and beyond the provision of resource guides that identify TGNC-affirming services (eg, electrolysis, endocrinologists, and beauticians) and steps for navigating government bureaucracy.[6,7] Although such guides and resources are certainly important to have and maintain, there may be more impactful ways to provide opportunities for learning and building cohesiveness. Inviting a guest speaker to discuss issues relevant to the group (eg, inviting an endocrinologist, sex therapist, or surgeon to facilitate a discussion about working with TGNC patients or inviting past group members to discuss their experiences in the therapy group) and organizing a group outing to participate in local advocacy work or fundraising are unique ways to foster knowledge and group cohesiveness.

Cohesiveness can also be fostered and maintained by creating a sense of group responsibility for assisting group members as they work toward their goals. The re-evaluation and assessment of progress toward goals ensure accountability of individual group members and compliance with competency D.3. One method to review progress toward goals and foster cohesiveness involves a group exercise wherein goals specified at the initial group meeting are revisited. In this exercise, group members are paired and each member of the dyad presents the goals of the other member and then offers his/her perspective on the progress that member has made toward achieving his/her respective goals. Feedback can then be solicited from the broader group. Group members making progress toward their goals have the opportunity to have their hard work acknowledged and reinforced. Group members who are not making progress toward their goals, despite having the means to do so, can receive feedback and encouragement from the group. Group members may share similar feelings of stagnation and be able to identify the skills they used to begin making progress.

This exercise can leave group members feeling vulnerable, especially if progress has been hindered by factors beyond the control of the group member. In such instances, it is important for the group to offer empathy and encouragement to the group member. A metaphor that may be offered in such instances is to draw a parallel to that of an airplane that is forced into a temporary holding pattern due to conditions on the ground. Thus, the leader attempts to instill hope at the possibility for circumstances to change in the future, while also encouraging the stymied/stuck group member to identify other goals that can be worked toward in the interim. A goal that serves this purpose and fosters cohesiveness is for a member to increase self-disclosure and interpersonal risk-taking within the group.

### Oppression and prejudice

TGNC group members inevitably discuss current or past experiences of oppression and prejudice. Competency D.5. specifies that group leaders must recognize how power, privilege, and oppression can have an impact on the group. Popular media and the Internet offer an ever-growing number of portrayals of TGNC people, and such portrayals can establish unrealistic expectations for what it means to be transgender. What the media sometimes fails to convey are the social and financial costs associated with being transgender and the debt that can be encumbered by TGNC people. Group leaders should be informed about these costs and should promote an open dialogue among group members about how financial privilege has an impact on the group process and individual members. In addition, the media and popular culture also seem to be giving greater attention to the prejudice that is experienced by many transgender people. Internalizing societal prejudice gives rise to internalized transphobia. Acknowledging institutionalized and internalized transphobia and how these processes have an impact on group members' abilities to disclose personal information within and outside the group is at the heart of competency D.9.

### Learned agency

One therapeutic tool that group leaders might consider using in TGNC groups to aid participants in fighting oppression is learned agency. Learned agency involves intentionally exhibiting behaviors that move clients toward their goals in the face aversive stimuli.[37] The learning histories of TGNC clients, especially as they relate to the direct expression of gender nonconforming behaviors, likely comprise invalidating and prejudiced experiences. In such instances, gender nonconforming behaviors may be punished to such an extent that not only is the behavior suppressed but also stimuli associated with the behavior become aversive. By providing information about basic learning principles and discussing the concept of learned agency, group leaders can assist group members in coming to recognize how their learning histories may have created learned roadblocks that prevent the members from attaining their goals, taking risks, and experiencing strong emotions. The case example of Shandra (a pseudonym) illustrates these dynamics:

> Shandra is an African American college student of Jamaican and Cameroonian ancestry in her early 20s who has recently joined a transgender-specific therapy group with the goal of becoming more comfortable with her identity as a trans woman. Shandra has 2 male roommates and only dresses in female clothes when she has the house to herself. Since the start of the group, Shandra has always arrived dressed in casual feminine clothing, wearing a wig and makeup. At the sixth group session, however, Shandra arrived in male attire. She explained that the previous night her roommate had come home unexpectedly, found her dressed in female clothing, and berated her verbally for her "perverted lifestyle." The group members provided support and sought to ensure that Shandra felt safe returning to her apartment. The group leader used this as an opportunity to discuss basic learning principles, including learned helplessness and learned agency, in an effort to highlight how avoidance of aversive stimuli can be reinforcing but maladaptive. Shandra expressed that she would like to continue to come dressed in female attire at future sessions but was reluctant to do so because she was afraid of having another unexpected and negative interaction with her roommate. Plans were made for Shandra to bring female clothing to the next session, arrive early, and use the clinic restroom to dress and apply makeup. Furthermore, Shandra was assisted by the group with role-plays to help her initiate a conversation with her roommate to discuss her gender identity and determine whether she and the roommate would be able to continue the current living arrangement without having future conflicts.

In this example, the group members were able to provide support to Shandra and help formulate concrete plans for overcoming the setback she experienced. Under ideal circumstances, this process can be carried out within the group setting, whereby reinforcement of learned agency occurs immediately. When this is not possible, it is essential that out-of-group activities be revisited in subsequent group sessions to reinforce success or provide support and problem solving, especially when group members' attempts to overcome their aversive learning histories are thwarted.

### Affect regulation

In addition to discussing learned agency, group leaders might consider teaching skills that promote affect regulation to help group members express strong emotions that may be associated with deeply personal or even traumatic experiences. Being able to express these emotions and discuss the associated experiences serves to enhance the sense of connectedness among group members, which in turn enhances cohesion. Goals for teaching affect regulation skills include the following: (1) identifying common emotional reactions to stress, (2) recognizing that multiple emotions can be experienced simultaneously and at varying levels of intensity, and (3) learning to implement stress reduction techniques to modulate physiologic arousal.[29] These goals can be achieved through the use of Socratic dialogue and by teaching skills that promote affect regulation, including diaphragmatic breathing, progressive muscle relaxation, and guided imagery. Affect regulation skills can also be used to help group members recognize their physiologic responses to stress and the connections between their cognitions, emotions, and behaviors.

### Cognitive interventions

Finally, cognitive coping/restructuring skills are likely beneficial in helping group members overcome problematic ways of thinking that come about as a result of living in a transphobic society. Austin and Craig[5] suggest a cognitive approach whereby transphobic beliefs about oneself are challenged by seeking out counterevidence. The group modality can be an especially powerful therapeutic tool, especially if there is diversity among the members regarding a particular belief. Thus counterevidence can often be elicited from the group to help challenge and erode negative self-beliefs.

In instances where transphobic cognitions persist despite efforts to challenge them with counterevidence, another approach involves drawing on a client's goals to promote cognitive flexibility.[29] In this context, thoughts are categorized not as "rational" or "irrational" but as "helpful," "neutral," or "unhelpful," depending on how the thought influences the group member's emotions and behaviors. The group leader works to help group members think about their experiences in ways that give rise to emotions and behaviors that move members toward their goals. When thoughts move members toward their goals via emotions and behaviors, those thoughts are considered "helpful." "Neutral" thoughts result in emotions and behaviors that neither move members toward or away from their goals, whereas "unhelpful" thoughts result in emotions and behaviors that move members away from their goals. A benefit of this simplified version of cognitive restructuring involves the ease with which it can be taught and understood within the group setting. This approach also incorporates the goals of the group member into the intervention and can offer an opportunity to discuss how members came to identify the goals that they are working toward. Such conversations can then easily be linked with a discussion of how the values of the group members influence their goals for the group.

### Termination

Termination provides an opportunity to again review each group member's goals and progress; it also offers a chance to identify new goals for the future (competency D.3.). In addition to reviewing progress within the group from the vantage point of each group member, group leaders can obtain additional data by using objective outcome measures. This is especially important in the group context, where nonspecific therapeutic factors, such as group cohesiveness, contribute to therapy outcomes and are likely more complex, relative to individual therapy. Thus, administering objective and validated psychotherapy outcome measures, such as the Outcome Questionnaire,[38] and psychotherapy process measures, like the Group Questionnaire,[39] are recommended. The use of these outcome assessments should be a minimum standard of practice for documenting group members' progress and informing future group therapy practice with TGNC clients. Through the combined use of objective and qualitative assessments as well as subjective feedback, group therapists might begin to answer critical questions pertaining to the efficacy of therapeutic interventions for TGNC clients. Group leaders might also be poised to better coordinate care with other professionals (competency D.12.), provide referrals for additional mental and/or physical health services (competency D.13.), and ensure continuity of care for group members as they continue working toward their goals.

## ADDITIONAL RECOMMENDATIONS FOR RESEARCH AND PRACTICE

This article highlights many practical issues related to the provision of group psychotherapy services for TGNC people. The following recommendations are offered in the spirit of advancing knowledge about how to meet the needs of this unique population.

First, psychotherapy researchers, including those developing group interventions, must ensure that their studies assess gender in ways that allow TGNC people to be identified. A recent systematic review of 232 randomized controlled trials with a combined sample size of more than 52,000 participants revealed that TGNC identities are not reported as demographic characteristics.[2] If these studies had reported TGNC identities, then it could have been possible to conduct secondary analyses to evaluate whether TGNC identification moderates treatment outcomes.

To remedy this problem, researchers can use a 2-step method to identify TGNC people. The Center of Excellence for Transgender Health Prevention[40] recommends asking, "What is your sex or current gender? (Check all that apply)" with the following response options: male; female; trans man; trans woman; genderqueer; and an additional category (followed by a request to "please specify" on a blank line). This question is followed by, "What sex were you assigned at birth?" with the response options of male; female; or declined to state. This method allows for the identification of persons who may be transgender but who do not specifically identify with a transgender label. It also allows for individuals to identify their sex in a multifaceted manner, thus capturing the complexity of the gender construct.[40]

Second, mental health professionals working with TGNC clients should have knowledge and understanding of the unique stressors that are experienced by transgender people that contribute to TGNC health disparities.[30,31] Scholars have demonstrated how Meyer's[41] minority stress model, which was originally developed to explain health disparities among gay men, generalizes to TGNC people.[31] Yet there may be unique stress processes (and mediators that link the experiences of stress to psychological distress) that are experienced by TGNC people that are not accounted for within this model.[30,42] Clinicians working with TGNC clients in group settings are ideally situated to help identify these processes; however, the knowledge must transfer from clinical to research settings and vice versa. Thus, there is a need for greater communication and collaboration between researchers and clinicians to bridge the research-practice divide. In bridging this divide, researchers and clinicians must also be mindful that not all forms of psychotherapy have been subjected to empirical evaluation, and many of these therapies may be beneficial for TGNC people, and thus their potential should not be discounted.

Finally, professional organizations that advocate for and advance the practice of group psychotherapy should consider how they might begin to promote research and scholarship pertaining to TGNC people. Such initiatives might include establishing scholarships or funding mechanisms to support research efforts specific to group work with TGNC populations. Other efforts might involve forming a subcommittee or working group to assess the state of the field and outline critical areas for future research. These organizations are also ripe for spearheading the development of best practices and practice guidelines that are specific to group work with TGNC clients. Finally, these organizations can engage in advocacy efforts to educate federal and private funding agencies about not only the impact of limited resources that are allocated to meeting the needs of this marginalized population but also the potential benefits that group psychotherapy has in promoting the health and well-being of TGNC people.

## SUMMARY

The ACA competencies highlight numerous important considerations for the provision of competent and affirmative group services to TGNC clients. Adherence to and embodiment of these competencies, in conjunction with a working knowledge of the guidelines and standards put forth by other professional organizations, should help enhance the quality of the services delivered to TGNC clients. Furthermore, scholarship on the topic of LGBT health suggests that the integration of specific interventions, such as psychoeducation, learned agency, affect regulation, problem solving, and cognitive coping, within the context of group psychotherapy for TGNC persons is desirable and effective.

Although the efficacy of many psychological interventions for use with TGNC clients has yet to be established, there is a small but growing body of scholarship dedicated to the provision of group psychotherapy services to this population,[6–8] and specific competencies that can help promote quality, transgender-affirmative care.[27] As the mental health professions make important efforts to highlight the needs of and challenges faced by TGNC people, the field is expected to move from simply writing about the experiences of group work with TGNC clients to actually empirically evaluating the effectiveness of interventions and developing interventions that demonstrate positive health and identity-related outcomes. As more training programs admit future scientists and practitioners with interests in transgender health, the future will only grow brighter. Until such time, clinicians are encouraged to reflect on and continue to enhance their competence for working with TGNC clients, to tailor evidence-based interventions where appropriate, and to remain mindful of the nonspecific factors that make the group modality a truly unique and powerful experience.

## REFERENCES

1. Flentje A, Bacca C, Cochran B. Missing data in substance abuse research? Researchers' reporting practices of sexual orientation and gender identity. Drug Alcohol Depend 2015;147:280–4.
2. Heck N, Mirabito L, LeMaire K, et al. Omitted data in randomized controlled trials for anxiety and depression: a systematic review of the inclusion of sexual orientation and gender identity. J Consult Clin Psychol 2016. http://dx.doi.org/10.1037/ccp0000123.
3. Pachankis J. Uncovering clinical principles and techniques to address minority stress, mental health, and related health risks among gay and bisexual men. Clin Psychol (New York) 2014;21:313–30.
4. American Psychological Association. Guidelines for psychological practice with transgender and gender nonconforming people. Am Psychol 2015;70:832–64.
5. Austin A, Craig S. Transgender affirmative cognitive behavioral therapy: clinical considerations and applications. Prof Psychol Res Pr 2015;46:21–9.
6. Dickey L, Loewy M. Group work with transgender clients. J Spec Group Work 2010;35:236–45.
7. Heck N, Croot L, Robohm J. Piloting a psychotherapy group for transgender clients: description and clinical considerations for practitioners. Prof Psychol Res Pr 2015;46:30–6.
8. Menvielle E, Rodnan L. A therapeutic group for the parents of transgender adolescents. Child Adolesc Psychiatr Clin N Am 2011;20:733–43.
9. Wampold B. The great psychotherapy debate. Mahwah (NJ): Lawrence Erlbaum Associates, Publishers; 2001.
10. Norcross J. Psychotherapy relationships that work. New York: Oxford University Press, Inc.; 2002.
11. Malyon A. Psychotherapeutic implications of internalized homophobia in gay men. J Homosex 1982;7:59–69.

12. Dworkin K, Pérez D, DeBord K. Handbook of counseling and psychotherapy with lesbian, gay, bisexual, and transgender clients. Washington, DC: American Psychological Association; 2007.

13. Singh A, Dickey L. In: Handbook of trans-affirmative counseling and psychological practice. Washington, DC: American Psychological Association; 2016.

14. Singh A, Dickey L. Implementing the APA guidelines on psychological practice with transgender and gender nonconforming people: a call to action to the field of psychology. Psychol Sex Orientat Gend Divers 2016;3:195–200.

15. Burlingame G, Fuhriman A, Mosier J. The differential effectiveness of group psychotherapy: a meta-analytic perspective. Group Dyn 2003;7:3–12.

16. Hogg J, Deffenbacher J. A comparison of cognitive and interpersonal-process group therapies in the treatment of depression among college students. J Couns Psychol 1988;35:304–10.

17. McDermut W, Miller I, Brown R. The efficacy of group psychotherapy for depression: a meta-analysis and review of the empirical research. Clin Psy Sci Prac 2001;8:98–116.

18. McRoberts C, Burlingame G, Hogg M. Comparative efficacy of individual and group psychotherapy: a meta-analytic perspective. Group Dyn 1998;2:101–17.

19. Herbst J, Jacobs E, Finlayson T, et al. Estimating HIV prevalence and risk behaviors of transgender persons in the United States: a systematic review. AIDS Behav 2008;12:1–17.

20. Yalom I, Leszcz M. The theory and practice of group psychotherapy. 5th edition. New York: Basic Books; 2005.

21. Lev A. Transgender emergence. Binghamton (NY): Haworth Clinical Practice Press; 2004.

22. Testa R, Jimenez C, Rankin S. Risk and resilience during transgender identity development: the effects of awareness and engagement with other transgender people on affect. J Gay Lesbian Ment Health 2014;18:31–46.

23. Sánchez F, Vilain E. Collective self-esteem as a coping resource for male-to-female transsexuals. J Couns Psychol 2009;56:202–9.

24. Yalom I, Houts P, Zimerberg S, et al. Prediction in improvement in group therapy: an exploratory study. Arch Gen Psychiatry 1967;17:159–69.

25. Freedman S, Hurley J. Perceptions of helpfulness and behavior in groups. Group 1980;4:51–8.

26. Coleman E, Bockting W, Botzer M, et al. Standards of care for the health of transsexual, transgender, and gender non-conforming people, version 7. Int J Trangend 2011;13:165–232.

27. Association of Lesbian, Gay, Bisexual, and Transgender Issues in Counseling. Competencies for counseling transgender clients. J LGBT Iss Coun 2010;4: 135–59.

28. Heck N, Flentje A, Cochran B. Intake interviewing with lesbian, gay, bisexual, and transgender clients: starting from a place of affirmation. J Contemp Psychother 2013;43:23–32.

29. Heck N. The potential to promote resilience: piloting a minority stress-informed, GSA-based, mental health promotion program for LGBTQ youth. Psychol Sex Orientat Gend Divers 2015;2:225–31.

30. Meyer I. Prejudice, social stress, and mental health in lesbian, gay, and bisexual populations: conceptual issues and research evidence. Psychol Bull 2003;129: 674–97.

31. Hendricks M, Testa R. A conceptual framework for clinical work with transgender and gender nonconforming clients: an adaptation of the minority stress model. Prof Psychol Res Pr 2012;43:460–7.
32. Chorplta B, Dalelden E, Weisz J. Identifying and selecting the common elements of evidence based interventions: a distillation and matching model. Ment Health Serv Res 2005;7:5–20.
33. Nezu A, Perri M. Social problem-solving therapy for unipolar depression: an initial dismantling investigation. J Consult Clin Psychol 1989;57:408–13.
34. Chorpita B, Weisz J. MATCH-ADTC: modular approach to therapy for children with anxiety depression trauma or conduct disorder. Satellite Beach (FL): Practice Wise, LLC; 2009.
35. Hayes S, Strosahl K, Wilson K. Acceptance and commitment therapy. 2nd edition. New York: Guilford; 2012.
36. Burlingame G, McClendon D, Alonso J. Cohesion in group therapy. Psychotherapy 2011;48:34–42.
37. Goodrich K, Luke M. Group counseling with LGBTQI persons. Alexandria (VA): American Counseling Association; 2015.
38. Lambert M, Lunnen J, Umphress K, et al. Administration and scoring manual for the outcome Questionnaire (OQ-45.2). Salt Lake City (UT): IHC Center for Behavioral Healthcare Efficacy; 1994.
39. Johnson J, Burlingame G, Olsen J, et al. Group climate, cohesion, alliance, and empathy in group psychotherapy. Multilevel structural equation models. J Couns Psychol 2005;52:310–21.
40. Sausa L, Sevelius J, Keatley J, et al. Policy recommendations for inclusive data collection of trans people in HIV prevention, care & services. San Francisco (CA): University of California; 2009.
41. Meyer I. Minority stress and mental health in gay men. J Health Soc Behav 1995; 36:38–56.
42. Hatzenbuehler M. How does sexual minority stigma "Get under the skin?" A psychological mediation framework. Psychol Bull 2009;135:707–30.

# Index

*Note:* Page numbers of article titles are in **boldface** type.

Psychiatr Clin N Am 40 (2017) 177–187
http://dx.doi.org/10.1016/S0193-953X(16)30091-0
0193-953X/17

# *Moving?*

## *Make sure your subscription moves with you!*

To notify us of your new address, find your **Clinics Account Number** (located on your mailing label above your name), and contact customer service at:

**Email: journalscustomerservice-usa@elsevier.com**

**800-654-2452** (subscribers in the U.S. & Canada)
**314-447-8871** (subscribers outside of the U.S. & Canada)

**Fax number: 314-447-8029**

**Elsevier Health Sciences Division**
**Subscription Customer Service**
**3251 Riverport Lane**
**Maryland Heights, MO 63043**

*To ensure uninterrupted delivery of your subscription, please notify us at least 4 weeks in advance of move.

Printed and bound by CPI Group (UK) Ltd, Croydon, CR0 4YY

07/10/2024

01040505-0015